My
Journey

Joseph Passaretti

ISBN 978-1-0980-9877-3 (paperback)
ISBN 978-1-0980-9878-0 (digital)

Christian Faith Publishing, Inc.
832 Park Avenue
Meadville, PA 16335
www.christianfaithpublishing.com

Printed in the United States of America

Dedication

T his book is dedicated to two of my dearest friends who lost their lives to cancer. Both were diagnosed around the same time that I was diagnosed.

Bob Gomes

Bob and I met in the late 1980's. He ran an after-market truck parts business in town and I would frequently purchase items from him or have him repair my trailer lights or the like. He was a very kind person always willing to help. Years later he hired me to assist with the accounting and tax work for his business. We fished together and attended hockey games together. Often we would meet at his boat and just sit and talk for a few hours, enjoying the evening sunsets near the water. Bob was diagnosed with cancer about a month before I was. His cancer was far more advanced though and was discovered when he was on vacation in Florida, with his wife, Denise. He ended up in the emergency room and was admitted to the hospital, where they found he had cancer. After a few weeks he ended up at Dana Farber in Boston and was doing very well for about two years. However, for some reason his body began to reject the treatments. He passed away about two weeks later. He was a true friend who had a significant influence on me. I miss him dearly and cherish the friendship we shared.

Wendy Costanza

I met Wendy in the mid 1990's in the course of my business where she was a salesperson for a national payroll company. During our first meeting it was as if we knew each other all our lives. We immediately became dear friends and she touched me in a way I cannot put into words.

Wendy was misdiagnosed for about a year before she ended up at Dana Farber. She fought the cancer for four years or so but for reasons I am not aware of, treatments no longer worked. Wendy was a fiercely independent woman who never complained about her treatments or how she felt. In the last few months of her life, we texted each other as she had trouble speaking. I still have all the texts and read them often. It brings me joy to know that SHE wrote these. She is one of the finest people I have ever met and I cherish our friendship.

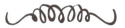

Contents

Special Thanks

First, I wish to express my sincere gratitude to my late mother, Barbara Passaretti, for being there for me throughout my life and for being the best mother anyone could have. She taught me to never stop looking forward and to always look for solutions to problems rather than being defeated by them. Her influence and teachings continue to guide me to this day. Special thank you to Dr. Jacob Laubach and his physician's assistant (who wishes to remain anonymous) for their dedication and continued support and for believing in me over the last four and a half years. Without them, I would not be writing these pages. To those who offered their support by sending cards of well wishes, calling to inquire of my progress, I thank you from the bottom of my heart. To my clients, who have also called the office to inquire of my status and progress, sent cards or stopped by just to offer support, I am forever grateful and humbled. Thank you for sticking by me through the difficult times. To my friends and family, specifically, Peter DeMasi, my dear friend from childhood for always staying connected and supporting me on almost a daily basis. To my cousin Dennis Passaretti, who has been a source of strength my whole life. And Ernie Almonte, who has been a true friend for many years and who has been so concerned about me and always offered to drive me to treatments. Thank you to Denise Gomes, who has continued to support me after losing her husband, Bob two years ago. Thank you Michael Canole, of the Rhode Island

Division of Taxation, for standing by me and understanding and helping all of the staff in my office when I was not available. To the late Maurice Anthony Lewis, the former Director of the Rhode Island Conservatory of Music, who taught me more about myself than he ever knew. To those who work in my office with me each and every day, without you I would never have been able to service our clients as well as we have. Special thank you to my dearest friends, the late Bob Gomes and Wendy Costanza, each of whom impacted me in such ways they never knew. I cherish their friendship and honor their memories. A special thank you to Captain Denny Dillon, Captain of the F/V Persuader II, out of Point Judith, Rhode Island, and to my uncle (on my wife's side) Louis Piccirilli, and our cousin Anthony Piccirilli, who frequently called and offered their help and support.

Most importantly I thank my wife, Linda, who had to endure all the pain of watching me fight the three cancers and for never losing faith in me. You are the light of my life.

Preface

This book is about my journey through life after being told I have cancer. The very word *cancer* makes people shiver and freeze in their tracks. Fortunately, I was never affected in that way but I certainly can understand how that one word could devastate someone. So I decided that I should tell my story to help those afflicted with cancer and those who care for these people. When someone is sick, whether it be cancer, Alzheimer's, stroke, or any other ailment, caregivers are affected as much as the patient is. I hope this book lends some inspiration and guidance to these patients and caregivers by the way I dealt with having cancer and facing death.

When I was diagnosed, I was examined at Brigham and Women's Hospital in Boston, Massachusetts, and treated at Dana-Farber Cancer Institute. At Dana-Farber, I was given the option to have treatments administered at Rhode Island Hospital. I declined because Dana-Farber is considered the best in the world and I wanted to be where I thought I would be exposed to the most experienced and knowledgeable doctors, nurses and back room people. I found exactly that.

This is not to degrade the professionalism or knowledge of those at other hospitals. The operations at Dana-Farber are world-class and this was very comforting. To know that all of the people there are so dedicated to their profession and not just there for a job—provided me with extreme confidence in everyone, including the phlebotomists, nurses, staff, and oncologists themselves. Everyone was on their game. Never was there a time when I felt alone or confused about the treatments, procedures, plan or the options. Never did I not feel I was in the best hands. Don't get me wrong, there were a couple of issues that took place with some lower level managers and employees. However, the actual doctors, nurses, and other people who treated me, performed tests, etc., were outstanding. I owe my life to them because they are so dedicated.

My wife, Linda, who is still the light of my life, was scared when we sat with Dr. Jacob Laubach at Dana-Farber for the first time. For her to hear the word *cancer* hurt me because it hurt her. I feel her pain. I think sometimes, more than she does. But she is strong and has faith in me so that made coping with the fact that I have cancer more manageable for her. I also believe that seeing me *not* defeated by the fact that I have cancer helped her cope and to witness everyday my adherence to what I stated to Dr. Laubach at that very first appointment, "I will do my utmost to keep normalcy in my life because normalcy helps a person heal."

I stand by this concept, which was drilled in me by my mother starting at a very early age. She would come into my bedroom and pull the covers off if I tried to sleep too late. If I was sick with a cold or just didn't feel good, she would insist I get up, shower and go do my normal things. And every time, I felt great! So I learned that this normalcy actually helps my body heal.

During that initial visit with Dr. Laubach, I was told that the cancer I have is rare and there is no cure. Treatments are limited, but Dr. Laubach stated he would do his best to treat me. He was somewhat set aback by my initial response to what he was telling us. He then stated to Linda that he does not believe I understood what he was saying. Linda and I looked at each other, and she responded, "Oh yes, he does. He is so far ahead of you in his thoughts and has already processed what you said."

I then responded to Dr. Laubach's concern as follows: I told him that we all are going to die. It is just a matter of when and how. While I am not interested in dying now, I needed his word that he would give me 150 percent effort and that I would rate him based upon only one metric. I stated, "If I live, you are the best; but if I die, you suck!" He was set aback but then realized that I was not joking. And to this day, I can honestly say he and his staff, especially his nurse practitioner, have given me 150 percent every day since January 2017.

After some discussion, Dr. Laubach mentioned that he was intrigued by my view of things. I told him the following, "I see this as a three-legged stool. The first leg is me. I will fight as hard as I can without any question. I will get up every day and do everything I always did because normalcy helps one heal. The second leg is you [Dr. Laubach] and your team. You must give me everything you have and more [150 percent] and never let up. Never become complacent. The third leg is God. If any one of these legs weakens, the stool falls. That is death, and death is unacceptable." He was stunned and stated that in all the years he has been practicing, he never heard it put so simply and honestly. He told me later that he uses this analogy with every new patient because it is so raw and from the gut, that it is extremely effective in offering hope to the new patients. Glad I could help!

There are so many people I want to recognize but can't because I simply don't know their names. So I will thank them as a group. These are the registration assistants, lab technicians, phlebotomists, parking attendants, cafeteria workers, x-ray technicians, various doctors and nurses who performed all the biopsies on me, pulmonary technicians who did the breathing tests, research assistants from the various studies I was participating in, research doctors who analyzed all the data taken from tissues, blood and urine (and whatever else they took from me) taken from my body for study, and all the other people I have not mentioned here who were a part, large or small, in taking care of me throughout this ordeal and who are *still* involved. All these people are from Brigham and Women's Hospital and Dana-Farber Cancer Institute in Boston, Massachusetts.

As for the doctors, each and every one of them have been superb, professional and 100 percent on their game. Dr. Emily Robinson, Dr. Jacob Laubach, Dr. Rodney Falk, and Dr. Anthony D'Amico. These are the people who have been steering the ship and keeping me on course from inception and continue to do so today. Without them, I believe the outcome of this disease would have been *much* more detrimental to my life because they pay attention and are proactive. Every time I meet with each, I always say, "Thank you," when we greet each other. They probably wonder why I do this, but it is because of their dedication to their profession and my well-being. I am so fortunate to have been in their care. And as I wonder how I met each, it occurs to me that each simply fell into place. Again, I am blessed to be in the care of each and every one of them.

One day one of my doctors asked me if I was afraid to die. "No," I responded. When asked why, I stated, "We are all going to die, it is just a matter of when and how." The doctor replied, "That is a very interesting way to look at it." To which I asked if he believed in a *God*. He stated he does, and that he is Catholic like me. Then I said, "We were taught to live by the teachings of God and to treat people the way we wish to be treated, to help others, to go about our daily lives and be conscious of what we do and try not to hurt others, etc." I asked if he prayed to God each day, and he said, "Yes." Then I asked him one question that summarizes the concept for me, "What the hell are you worried about? If you live as God teaches us and you help others," which he does, "you will go to heaven and get your wish."

The look on his face was astounding. It told of a realization he just experienced that is so simple, so raw that it hit home. He expressed this to me. It doesn't matter if you are Catholic, Protestant, Muslim, Buddhist, Jewish, or any other identified religion. It matters that you live by *your god's* teachings and help others. I look at life this way: each minute we are a boat traveling down a river. The boat makes a wake in its path. We must be aware of the effects of this wake on others and ensure that the wake does not injure anyone on shore, or in the water.

I can recall when Linda and I were dating back in the early 1980s. We drove to the Town Beach of Narragansett, Rhode Island, to be by the water. As we drove, we came to a roundabout, and a man was riding a bicycle, and he fell near the sidewalk. He must have hit some sand or something. Immediately and instinctively, I pulled over and got out of the car to help the man. He was so grateful that someone helped him. As I reentered the car, Linda was staring at me. I asked, "What?" Her response told it all. She said nothing. This was a defining moment for me that I never mentioned to anyone. You see, I learned something that morning, that while I always *thought* of such a response to someone in need, the immediate intrinsic reaction proved that this is inside of me. *That* is why Linda was so amazed. She realized this, and I believe it taught her something about herself as well. She realized that I never thought about reacting this way, it just came to me. And *that* is the teaching of God inside of me. Throughout my life, I would experience this in several areas of my life, from things that happened while fishing, or with interns at my office or with nature too.

In the early 1990s a barge carrying crude oil landed on a beach in South Kingstown, Rhode Island, spilling thick toxic oil into the water and on the beaches, into estuaries, etc. It was a major event. I recall that the authorities were on television showing how birds were covered in oil and could not fly. So they were picking up the birds and washing them, and I just had to help. So I left the office and took a few days on the beach in January helping with picking up oil-covered birds, bringing them to an area of the beach where the authorities were collecting and washing or treating them and went off to continue. Afterwards, I recall thinking about the event and realized my reaction was spontaneous. I never thought about it, but the need to respond to this just happened. Again, I believe this was God speaking through me. Don't misread my intention here. I am not applauding myself but simply telling about how the power of one's God can make things happen without one even realizing it until sometime later.

So following is my story of the almost daily account of the life I have led since being diagnosed with cancer in January 2017. I begin with some historical content. The information provided is factual and based on my own experiences. The test result numbers published here are actual reports from my record at Dana-Farber and Brigham and Women's Hospital. They are here to illustrate the changes in my test numbers and the representations of the information I have outlined in text.

Early Years

It all started in January 1959 in Providence, Rhode Island. Born to Enrico (Henry) and Barbara (Vita) Passaretti, we lived on Federal Hill, a section of Providence where Italian American families settled from the old country and the Italian mob ruled but took care of the civilians. The youngest of three, I was always extremely close to my mom. She was the wind in my sails instilling values and confidence in every stage of my life. To this day, her teachings guide me through all things in my life.

My brother and I attended Holy Ghost School and were altar boys at the Holy Ghost Church. The pastor at that time, Father Parente, was a very scary man. He was strict and scared the daylights out of me. I can recall I was assigned the task of ringing the bell at certain times during the Mass. Kneeling on the marble altar and being skin and bones as I was so small, my knees would hurt. So I would fidget, and the bell would ring at the wrong time. Father Parente would glance over my way with disapproval, and his look would make me shake, so the bell would go off again. If looks could kill, I would be dead several times over. He would later try to talk with me, and I would explain my dilemma, but he wouldn't hear of it. So we kept on going that way for a long time. My brother was scared for me and would ask, "Why can't you stay still?" Looking back, this was comical. Imagine being a parishioner in the pews and watching this going on. Hearing the bell at the wrong times and trying not to laugh during Mass.

When I was five years old, Mom told me and my brother, Henry, who was six, to "pick a musical instrument because you are going to learn how to play it." I picked the guitar and Henry the drums. It was *great*. Two young kids being allowed to pursue a dream of playing music. We thought we were rock stars. Then came the reality—mom signed us up for music lessons! I can recall my first teacher being Ed Di Pippo on Federal Hill in Providence. I used to have to climb a flight of stairs to the second floor to the practice room where my lessons were taught. Mr. Di Pippo commented once that he always knew when I was coming because he could hear the body of the guitar hitting the steps as I climbed them. You see, the instrument was bigger than I was. Being a short and very tiny person, I could not lift the guitar high enough to clear the stairs. It was amusing to Mr. Di Pippo, but I was just trying to make the stairs for lessons.

After Mr. Di Pippo, I studied with several private teachers, but at the age of twelve, Mom realized that I was very interested in the study and took me to the Rhode Island Conservatory of Music on Benefit Street in Providence. We met the director, Maurice Anthony Lewis, on a Saturday morning. After some discussion, Mr. Lewis asked me to play something on an acoustic guitar that he had at the studio and to read and play a few bars from a written manuscript. Mr. Lewis accepted me to the conservatory that morning. I recall being so excited that I couldn't sleep that night.

I studied at the conservatory under Mr. Lewis for several years. This study taught me more about myself than the music. You see, the discipline of the formal study of music allowed me to find my strengths and weaknesses, and to overcome the latter. This strength was an example of the inner reliance that we were taught at such a young age. I think that one of the reasons I excelled in this study was because it allowed me to experience a real-life situation where the very thing mom taught me was happening, and I could see the success in it. Strength from inside.

Another example of the result of this inner strength occurred when I was nine years old, and I caught my right hand in the blades of a lawn mower, chopping off three fingers and my thumb. Running into the house with my hanging fingers, Mom instinctively wrapped my hand and the severed fingers on ice in a kitchen towel and directed Dad to get me to the hospital. The three of us were in Dad's station wagon racing down High Service Avenue, Smith Street and Chalkstone Avenue to Roger Williams Hospital, Providence, Rhode Island. Most people would have called an ambulance, but Mom always believed when necessary one can only rely on his/herself. Time being of the essence, there was no waiting for someone to come to us, so we went to them.

After several hours of surgery, my fingers were once again a part of my hand, thanks to the extremely talented late Dr. Howard Sturim. I would find out thirty years later that Dr. Sturim was merely an intern at that time, and here I come with one of the worst things he would face. He told me during a chance meeting years later that he was more scared than I, and that this helped shape his future. Amazing!

It seems that even he would be brought to understand that his own self-reliance is the most effective and important strength in times of trauma or any major event. We all face some kind of traumatic events in our lives. The outcome is, in my opinion, a function of the strength one possesses that allows him/her to deal with it.

After leaving Federal Hill, we moved to Johnston, Rhode Island, for a short time and then to North Providence. This move was not planned however. One Saturday morning, my mom took us roller skating in Georgiaville in the Esmond section of Smithfield, Rhode Island. I cannot recall the name of the skating rink, but we skated. And then as we left, Mom got lost, and we ended up in a very nice neighborhood in the Woodhaven section of North Providence. Not knowing where in the world we were, Mom heard music coming from a house and decided to stop and ask for directions. The music was coming from a speaker mounted on the outside of the house. We were amazed as we never saw such a thing before. It was an intercom system, one of the first made and installed in this house.

Mom rang the bell, and a woman came to the door. The intent was to ask for directions back to Centredale in North Providence,

Rhode Island, but the woman invited us in. My brother and I were gazing at this beautiful house, which looked enormous because there was no furniture. So Mom inquired about the house. The woman responded that her husband just completed building the house, and she was cleaning it in order to put it up for sale. Mom asked for a tour, and the woman was more than accommodating. After the tour, Mom and the woman came to handshakes, and we were moving out of Johnston and into North Providence's Woodhaven Manor section. Now Mom had to tell Dad. This was not unusual because she often went ahead and entered into business deals and later would tell him, and he would be okay with it. She did this with two commercial buildings she purchased for his jewelry business and came back to inform him he was no longer renting. She had an eye for real estate and an acumen for business, and he knew it so he never argued the point.

I attended North Providence High School where I was not exactly a model student. You see, both the principal and vice principal were friends of my dad, so I was treated quite liberally: allowed to skip classes without consequences, leave school grounds to run errands for the vice principal, and other things. As a student, I thought this was great. What young kid wouldn't?

After graduation in 1978, and after a short and very eye-opening stint at my dad's jewelry shop, I was still studying at the Rhode Island Conservatory of Music, and in 1979, Mom suggested I go to college. More on this later.

One of the major influences on my inner strength is my belief in God. I know some do not believe, and that is okay with me. But my strong belief is essential to the inner strength I have found that has allowed me to face those traumatic situations in my life. And there were many more than stated in these pages. I will not bore you with these but they affected my siblings' lives and my parents' as well. I had to deal with these things alongside my mother, and that required a significant sense of inner balance and strength. I never would have possessed this strength without the guidance of my mother, my belief in God, and the formal study of music to teach me about myself.

I met Linda in 1980 in what I call a divine intervention. My friend Tom was trying to secure a date with a girl named Donna. So one night he called and asked me to accompany him to a local disco club in Providence, Rhode Island, where Donna was supposed to be. I was sick with a fever and the flu, so I was reluctant to go, but Tom and I were very good friends; and still are, so I agreed. When we arrived, I stated I would be sitting in the back of the facility at a table near the windows. So that is where I parked myself. The windows were opened because it was August, and a nice breeze was coming in off the bay. With a pitcher of water, I was just fine.

After about fifteen minutes, a girl I have known for many years saw me and asked what the heck I was doing there. I explained the circumstances to her. You see, I was *not* a clubber—or as I refer to people who frequented these facilities—a lounge lizard. She knew this and was shocked to see me there. I was basically a fish out of water. I did, however, enjoy listening to the music, though the genre was not my style. So we sat and talked for some time and out of nowhere came Linda. It appears they were there together with other girls, and since we were in the back of the room, no one could really see us. Linda was apparently looking all over for her friend but couldn't find her. Upon finding us, Linda stated she was looking for her friend for an hour. Her friend told her she was sitting, talking with me, and the first words to me out of Linda's mouth were, "So you are the—[Italian for big mouth or talker], who monopolized my friend." *Boom!* Lightning struck! I asked our friend who the hell this girl is, and she introduced us. That was it! Something happened at her very first words.

My friend Tom struck out, and as we walked to the car, he was kicking stones in the road from disappointment. You see, Donna was not even there so he was so disappointed. I felt bad but I disclosed to him at that point, "Tom, I met my wife tonight." He said, "What?" I repeated it and said, "I don't know, but I need to find out everything I can about Linda." So I went on a mission to find out everything I could about her: where she lives, what kind of car she drives, license plates, etc. I needed to find her. I made numerous calls to friends and gathered all I could about her, and each weekend I would show up at the club she and her friends were at that night. They went to discos throughout Rhode Island and Boston, Massachusetts, as that was the "thing" then.

Linda never knew how I found her each time, but years later I told her that many of the people at the clubs were friends who were bouncers. I met them in either the music business or through the martial arts arena, where I spent some time training with the late great George Pesare and my cousin Dennis Passaretti, who is known throughout the world as one of the top martial artists of all time. I gave them her plate number and make of her car and asked that they call me if she showed up, and they all did. Sometimes, someone I knew would be at the particular club she would be at and they would call me. *Surprise!* I would say. She played hard to get, but one day I stated to her that she may win the battle but I would win the war.

The lightning strike was instant love. I still cannot tell you what happened because it hit me so fast, but I still feel that same feeling each and every day. I truly believe that she and I were destined to meet and be together, and I thank God every day for Linda.

In 1987, Linda and I were married at Blessed Sacrament Church in Providence, Rhode Island. My brother, Henry, was my best man and I can recall standing with him near the foot of the altar waiting as Linda and her dad were walking down the aisle. The church was so large and there were so many people standing and watching Linda come down the aisle that Henry and I couldn't see her for some time. And then she appeared, and as my eyes saw her for the first time, in that beautiful white dress, my knees buckled and Henry saw this and grabbed me by the arm to hold me up. I have never seen such a beautiful sight than Linda in that dress walking down the aisle with her handsome dad.

When her dad (his nickname is Suny because of his perpetual smile) handed her off to me, we walked up the altar to where the priest was waiting for us. We had a large "unity" candle on a tall pedestal on the altar and we were to light this candle together as a sign of eternal unity. So we approached and did this. During rehearsal, I was told to turn away from the candle when blowing out the long matchstick. Easy, right? Nope! I blew out the stick and the candle together. Right there, Linda looked at me with anger in her eyes. I am not sure anyone even saw this, but it happened; and for the first time as a married man, the first thing my new wife did was scold me. Still going on today. I have often said that if Linda is not scolding me for something, I know I am in trouble because that would be an indication she no longer cares. So, as I see it as long as I am in trouble, I'm good!

My father-in-law, Suny, and I actually met before I ever met Linda. Some of his friends were people I knew from when I was younger, and I would run into him occasionally. So when I met Linda and went to her house for the first time, there he was. As we saw each other, I asked, "What are you doing here?" His response was, "The better question is what are *you* doing here?" That was the beginning of a wonderful relationship, one that I still cherish to this day. Over the years, we would fish and attend game dinners together or just hang out. We were friends as well as in-laws. I am truly honored to know him. He once told me that I am the son he never had. What an honor! A gentleman, he would seldom raise his voice or enter into conflict. His face seemed to always have a smile on it, and his willingness to help people was awesome.

Over the years, we grew closer and would talk alone about things that I never have disclosed and will take with me to the grave. Suny suffered with Alzheimer's disease and passed away in September 2019. Toward the last several months of his life, he didn't know anyone's name but still had that smile on his face and was always happy to see everyone. He was especially close to Linda and when she walked in the room, his face lit up. She addressed him with such delicacy and love it was heartwarming to witness. He responded too! It is evidence that their bond was unbreakable. Though she is devastated by his passing, she finds comfort that one day they will be with each other again.

Linda is the light of my life. She brings me such inner joy and peace, and she keeps me grounded. She is the levelheaded one of the pair. You see, I am somewhat impulsive and will do just about anything on a spur-of-the-moment. She, however, is far more reserved and contained. It works well for us, and the spontaneity was something that helped me win her over when we were dating. It kept her surprised many times.

After the wedding reception held at the Alpine Country Club in Cranston, Rhode Island, Linda and I went on our honeymoon. One of my clients owned a limousine service and he picked us up and drove us to T. F. Greene Airport in Warwick, Rhode Island. We flew to Los Angeles and went on a cruise of the Mexican Riviera. Ports of call were Mazatlán, Porta Vallarta, and other beautiful stops. Linda said we had a great time. I don't recall any of it! The only thing I recall was being in a glass bottom boat and wishing Henry was with us so that he could see it.

My memory of the honeymoon seems to have been erased by the tragic event of my brother's death. You see, two days before the end of our honeymoon, Linda and I were in Marina del Rey, California, sleeping at a hotel room when the telephone rang at 3:00 a.m. local time. It was my mother's brother. He informed me that my beloved brother passed away by an industrial accident. This single event erased my memory of our honeymoon. Immediately I asked to speak with my mother, who did get on the telephone to speak with me. She was very upset and told me she had to see my brother. She knew that somehow I would make this happen. I didn't know how but I asked her to give me a couple of hours and I will call her back with the required protocol to see him at the morgue.

It was only 6:00 a.m. back in Rhode Island, so I could not call anyone immediately. However, around 8:00 a.m. I began calling powerful local people in Rhode Island and was able to speak directly with the Rhode Island medical examiner. I stated to the ME that if she did not allow this to happen, she would have another body there in her morgue—Mom's. She would die of a broken heart and with too many questions. She stated that it was not something that was ordinarily done but if someone would accompany Mom, she would allow it. I agreed, but stated that Mom needs to be alone with Henry in the room. The person accompanying her would have to wait outside. She agreed.

Several hours later, Mom called me at the hotel in Marina Del Rey, and I asked her if she was now okay. She said yes. I never asked any other questions. This was a mother-son thing that I did not have the cerebral or inner capacity to comprehend. It can only be understood by a parent, which I was not. But I understood the need as I could hear it in Mom's voice. To this day, I am so happy I could pull through for her. She never asked how I made this happen because it did not matter. The effort was not to be confused with the result!

We arrived at T. F. Greene Airport from our honeymoon the next day on an emergency flight. I do recall when Linda's dad picked us up at the airport that day. His face was so somber I can still see it in my mind. This is a man who had a perpetual smile on his face, and to see it gone demonstrated the pain he felt for my brother, me, and especially his daughter.

Suny drove us to my mom's house, and I do recall seeing my mom waiting at the door. Her little body, all four feet one inch of it, was behind the glass door; and as I walked up the three steps to the door, she hugged me. Our bond was strong. I asked if she is okay, and she was remarkably so. She too possessed that inner strength she taught me to have. Here is a woman who just lost her middle child, oldest son, and she was poised, aware, and never flinched. Sure, she was devastated but her inner strength provided her with the power to move forward even in such tragic times. After she was able to meet with my deceased brother, she emerged stronger and at peace. One thing that I recall realizing at that moment was that the teachings of inner strength were not theoretical but I saw first-hand that it works in practice. I was so impressed by her ability to be strong and to be at peace with herself, and the fact that Henry was gone, it impacted me in great ways.

Another Experience
with Death

My brother's death was the most devastating I ever dealt with along with that of my mom. But in 1979, I experienced my first bout with death of a person very close to me. Mr. Lewis passed away suddenly during a performance at a local restaurant. He suffered a heart attack at the piano. I received a call from his family the day after the death, and I was devastated.

I took time off from the conservatory where I was now an assistant teacher writing scores for other students and filling in for Mr. Lewis. He asked if I would be interested in teaching full time, and we agreed I would take a few weeks off and think about it. I never did get a chance to speak with him again. Once I received that call that he passed away, I did not play an instrument for almost ten years. Again I was devastated.

Being somewhat lost from the shock of it all, I was working at my father's jewelry shop where I was unable to perform most of the work on any of the machines. Dad took me off the polishing wheels and put me on the degreasing cleaning machine where I would lower trays of polished jewelry into the machine and spray them with hot trichlorethylene. The problem was the fumes would make me so high, I couldn't function. So mom suggested one day that I go home and change clothes and go to the local community college. She said that I could enroll in business courses and that before long I would find my subject. Once again, she was right. Within one month, I was finding myself engrossed in the subject of accounting. Everything seemed to work because everything always had to balance. So I majored in accounting at Bryant College, now Bryant University, in Smithfield, Rhode Island.

Bryant was another major teaching event in my life. The study of accounting taught me more about myself than accounting. In fact, the discipline of music seems to have helped me understand the intricacies of the study of accounting. There are many historical events that I learned about during the study of music and that of accounting at Bryant College. In particular, during my study of music, I learned that Beethoven was deaf but could feel the beat of the music by the vibrations of each note. This takes a tremendous amount of self-awareness and confidence, and we are the benefactors of Beethoven's abilities through his music. To quote Langston Hughes, "Exactitude in tiny matters is the very sole of discipline."

You Have Cancer

January 23, 2017, was a routine day with a doctor's appointment at 9:00 a.m. in the Foxboro, Massachusetts, location of Brigham and Women's Hospital. My doctor is Emily Robinson, a nephrologist who had been watching my increased protein levels in my urine for a couple of years. During our visit, we talked about my status. Remember this was prediagnosis. We had no idea at this point of any cancer. Routinely, she ordered urine samples and blood work.

I had another nephrologist before Dr. Robinson. This man was from Rhode Island and practiced at Rhode Island Hospital. After two visits I decided this man was not for me. He was very nice, and he was certainly qualified. However, he had a cavalier attitude about him and a demeanor that he was the focus of attention. Excuse me, but you work for *me* remember? I asked for my files and left for Emily Robinson. I firmly believe that I was guided by something much bigger than me and that had this change not have been made, and at the time it was made, I would be dead today.

The next morning, she called me from her home, where she was working that day, and stated she read my labs and suspected I have two types of cancer, multiple myeloma and amyloidosis, a rare form of cancer that impacts the organs due to proteins attaching to the organ and killing it. My response was, "Okay, what do we do?" She responded, "Exactly!" and stated she scheduled a kidney biopsy for the next day. I was to arrive at the main facility of Brigham and Women's Hospital in Boston for 5:00 a.m. I did.

The biopsy was nothing too exciting. I requested no Novocain because that seems to have a long-lasting effect on my brain, making me lack lucidity for about two to three months at least. The doctor performing the biopsy was stunned to see that I requested this. He said he was going to insert a probe into my lower hip area and several inches into me with about four inches into the kidneys, take some samples, and be done with it. Then the other side. So I asked him how long he would have the probe in me, and he stated about one minute each. My response was that two minutes (three samples each kidney) of pain is much less to tolerate than months of fogginess. He understood and proceeded to perform the biopsy, which in fact revealed exactly what Dr. Emily Robinson thought. Multiple myeloma and amyloidosis. She already had me scheduled to see the next doctor, who would be a pivotable person in my treatment, recovery, and prospect of living a reasonably long life. His name is Dr. Jacob Laubach, chief of Oncology for my type of cancer at Dana-Farber Cancer Institute.

You see, Emily Robinson saved my life (she denies this, but I know better) because she cared and paid attention. Something that is routine in Boston, but unfortunately, not everywhere. Money is no issue there as it is at some institutions. I never had to worry about what was covered by insurance because I was entered into research studies that would contribute tests, drugs, etc. that would not be covered by all medical insurances. This is what separated the men from the boys. Dana-Farber is world class, and the objective is to treat and save lives, not money. I was incredibly impressed and blessed to have been introduced to Jacob Laubach. Again, had I not met Emily Robinson, I would probably be dead today.

The first day I went to Dana-Farber, I was asked to see another doctor at the Brigham and Women's Hospital, Dr. Rodney Falk. He is my amyloid cardiologist. You see, the cancer infiltrated my heart so Dr. Falk was called in. This is where I was asked to participate in the first study. The research assistant and research doctor told me that the results of their research probably would not benefit me (it was thought I would not live too long) but may help others in the future. I agreed as I saw this as a no-brainer. All I needed to do was answer questions, have urine and blood work done, and take certain tests that the research required. You see, the consensus was that I would probably not live too long as there was not much treatment and *no* cure for the amyloidosis.

What I learned later in time was that these tests were being used as part of my treatments and afforded the doctors information they otherwise would not have been able to obtain because insurance would not cover the specific tests, etc. So it turns out I *did* receive a benefit from participating in the research studies. My understanding is that they have also come up with a few new drugs to address amyloidosis since I was diagnosed. Some that were developed, I am told, was a result of the research having being done.

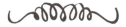

Treatments

There are many myths regarding the treatments for cancer. In my case, there was no nausea, vomiting, loss of my hair, although there was a thinning of hair, but that could also be attributed to age. I was blessed throughout the process. The major side effect of my chemo came in the form of sudden exhaustion. I would be perfectly fine and energetic, and without notice or any eventuality, I would suddenly be unable to function. This would force me to pull over and rest if I was driving, or if working at the office, simply sit back in my chair, close my eyes and rest for ten minutes. Then as sudden as it appeared, it vanished. This would happen mostly in the late afternoon, say around 3:00 p.m. to 4:00 p.m. However, it usually only happened in the afternoon after a morning treatment and the next day or two. After that, I was fine again.

In order to hedge against infection and to work to stimulate the chemo drugs, etc., I was given Dexamethasone (Dex) the day of treatments. This really had the most noticeable impact on me. This would make my heart race up to 150 bpm at rest. I own a Samsung Galaxy watch and would sometimes wear it to bed as it would periodically take my heart rate. While sleeping on several occasions, my heart would beat up to 150 bpm and sometimes higher when awake. The doctors reduced the dosage of Dex to a more reasonable level after several months, and it was *much* better. I would reach ninety-five at rest instead of one hundred fifty, and this would usually subside in a few days.

One of the most important things to do when receiving chemo treatments is to drink *plenty* of water. I can recall drinking up to one gallon of water a day because I felt like the chemo was sucking the fluids out of my body. The lab work focused on the creatinine levels as a guide to my levels of fluid. Many times this level would indicate I was not drinking enough. *What!* Gallons of water and this is not enough? Turns out when I took the labs it was early morning and I had not yet had sufficient fluids to lower the levels for a good reading. I figured out that I could wake up earlier and begin the intake of water earlier and the levels came down. Creatinine is a level of kidney function as well. It is important that this level be sufficient or the drugs could harm the kidneys.

Treatments would last about an hour to two hours, depending on the drugs given to me at that time and the dosages as well. Preparation time is the thing that takes time. Blood work for labs, insert the catheter in my arm (I was not given a port in my main artery as my veins were considered very healthy), then a shot of Velcade, which is another chemo drug. This was usually given in the stomach at Dana-Farber. One time I had to move my treatment day from a Thursday to a Wednesday as there was a major issue at the office. Since Wednesday was not my normal day, I was assigned a nursing staff that was not my normal staff. You see, at Dana-Farber the patient always has the same nurses as they get to know you inside and out.

The new head nurse told me that she was to give me the shot of Velcade. This is normally administered in the stomach and leaves the patient with a burn about the size of the palm of your hand. It lasts for about two to three weeks. So because of the burn, or bruise as they refer to it, they need to move around the torso so as not to administer over a current bruise. After I responded to the nurse's inquiry about whether or not I am bruised, she stated that she could administer the drug in the thigh. I was somewhat surprised at this suggestion because I thought they could only administer in the stomach. She went on to explain the reasoning for the thigh, and I felt comfortable with it, but told her to go ahead and administer in the stomach. She did. I even made a comment that I will not put on these pages, but was genuinely concerned about being exposed in front of someone I didn't even know. The nurse was amused by this because of the sincerity of the comment and began to laugh about it.

You see, the professionals at Dana-Farber are just that—professionals. Their days are filled with "bad" things, people with cancer. Some doing well and others not so well. Some even moving to death at a rapid pace. The response I rendered and spoke of was received very well because it was considered outside the norm and real. I was not being fresh with her just telling the truth and it was real. She inherently understood this and considered this a sort of comic relief moment. Most welcome over the normal critical, hard work, and negativity they see all day long.

When I told Linda about this, she was appalled. "You didn't!" she said. When I explained the situation to her and that this was my heartfelt reaction, she just looked at me and sighed and shook her head. I went on to explain to her the reaction of the nurse, and while she was relieved, she still did not like that I responded this way. Maybe I should have refrained from the comment, but this is what was in my thoughts at that moment. Linda always says that I don't have to say *everything* I am thinking!

Amazing Events

I have made numerous visits to Dana-Farber Cancer Institute for treatments, tests, consults, and other reasons. During these meetings, I met so many incredible people: doctors, nurses, administrators, and so many more. Two such visits truly stand out because of the people I met. I will change the names in order to protect privacy.

I was sitting in the waiting room one afternoon on a day I was not usually there. As I mentioned earlier, my original appointment for treatment was for Wednesday but something came up at my office and I asked to receive treatments a day early. So I was sitting in the waiting area, and about two o'clock from me was a woman with a young girl. Reading a magazine, I notice on occasion the young girl would look at me. When I looked back at her, she quickly looked away as if to hide something or not let me know she was staring. After about three or four times, I asked her name.

"Jill," she stated. "What's yours?"

I said, "Joe."

She asked, "What are you doing here?"

I responded that I was waiting to receive treatments. So I asked, "What are you doing here?"

She said, "I am waiting to get treatments too."

Meanwhile, her mom was listening to this entire conversation. Then she asked, "You're sick?"

I responded, "Yes."

"How come you don't look sick?" she asked.

"I don't know. How come *you* don't look sick?" I asked.

She replied "I don't?"

I said, "No."

At that point, there was nothing said for about a minute. I could see she was thinking because she stared at the floor and was contemplating something. So I snapped my fingers and said, "I know why we don't look sick."

"*Why?*" she asked.

I said, "God made only so many perfect people. The rest don't have blue eyes?" (We both have blue eyes.)

She laughed, and her mom laughed. Suddenly she began to cry intensely. I was so nervous because I had no idea what I did to hurt her. At that point, the medical assistant called her in for treatments, and she sprinted to the door as if to get out of sight. There I was wondering what the hell just happened.

I learned later that Jill turned eighteen a couple of days earlier, and up to this day, she was very reluctant to receive her treatments. Her parents had to pull rank as she was a minor. If she refused today's treatments, then no one could do anything about it. I did not know this at that time. You see, I am told, sometimes young people who are diagnosed with cancer oftentimes think they are different from their peers; they think they look different as well. Sometimes they do look different. But not in this case.

It turns out that Jill started to cry because, as I found out, she realized I don't even know her and recognized she looks normal and great. The crying was from relief and not pain. Someone who was familiar with this matter later stated, "You saved a life today."

Imagine I was at Dana-Farber on a day I was not supposed to be there, and this happens. What are the odds? My only conclusion is that we were both meant to be there. I truly believe God put us there so that we could meet, and the result is clear.

The second major event was when I met a man who was so miserable it was actually funny. Here is what happened: I was sitting in the treatment waiting area and saw this man sitting across from me. We will call him Bill. I went and sat next to him and asked how he was doing. His response was, "How does it look like I'm doing?"

I was set aback. I introduced myself, and his response was, "So what!"

Okay, now I knew I was sitting next to a *very* miserable person. About a minute of silence, he asked me what I was doing there. I told him I was waiting to receive treatments. He too was waiting for treatment. I asked what type of cancer he has, and he told me, but I just cannot recall the name of it or where it was. I guess I was so stunned by his initial response I was half-listening. Then he asked what type of cancer I have. I replied, "I have two types: multiple myeloma and amyloidosis."

He replied, "Oh, that's bad!"

I replied, "Thanks, Bill."

We began talking about treatments and other things, and he said he was so tired from the treatments he had to stop working. So I asked what he did for work. "I am an accountant," he replied.

I thought he was going to say construction, fisherman or some other laborious position. "*What*? An accountant? You mean you can't sit your skinny little ass in a chair and work numbers and make decisions?"

To that he replied, "F— you!"

I said, "Well f— you too, Bill!"

Then we laughed together. He asked me what I do, and I simply pulled out a business card and handed it to him. "No way!" he said.

"Yep, I am an accountant."

I then proceeded to explain my approach to the entire cancer thing. I said that I believe having stopped working was the worst thing to do because normalcy helps one heal. I told him that his body is going through enough changes and turmoil, and that to change what is normal in his life was only going to make matters worse. He asked if I am still working, and I told him I work every day. If I get tired, I told him how I deal with it.

The next week, I saw Bill in the lobby, and he was dressed in a suit. I said "Bill, nice suit."

He said, "I went back to work, and I feel so much better."

I was crying again. I don't cry, but these two events put me to tears. I was so happy to hear that. He said he feels he has purpose again. I encouraged Bill to keep it up. When that sudden exhaustion comes upon him, I said, "Take a snooze at your desk. Or do as I do, eat a couple of dark chocolate candies. They worked wonders for me."

Operate My Business

D r. Emily Robinson called with the news of protein in my urine on January 23, 2017, and this was the beginning of the tax-filing season, January to April 15, and hundreds of corporate and individual clients rely on our office to advise them regarding taxes and prepare their returns for filing.

The next day or so, I sat down with my staff and explained the situation. I instructed them that I could not sit with clients this tax season due to the low immune system resulting from the treatments. Most of my clients have been with me for at least twenty years and are accustomed to sitting with me during tax time. It is as much a social event as a tax filing and planning event.

My wife, Linda, brought up a concern about not meeting with these people after so many years. She stated that they would not appreciate it and feel that I was disregarding them. To this I responded that her concern is valid. However, we would inform every client about my cancer and the reasons I could not sit with them. I expressed my feeling that my relationship with these people goes far beyond our work. I believed that it would be disrespectful *not* to tell them, and this would demonstrate that they are just what they're not—simply a financial transaction. I felt they would under-stand, and 95 percent did. The other small percentage bailed out because they probably thought I would die and they would need to find someone else anyway.

The overwhelming support from my clients was humbling. They were told of my situation and participated in prayer sessions at churches, sent us cards, and called on a frequent basis inquiring of my progress. All the people who stood by me proved that in business, there is far more than just a financial transaction. There is a bond that only became evident to me upon sickness. I thank every one of my clients who stood by me. Needless to say, we had the best year to that point in the history of my practice. Unbelievable!

I also want to express that some of the department leaders at the Rhode Island Division of Taxation were also *very* supportive and caring. Michael Canole especially proved that he is a true friend. His understanding and caring was incredible. A remarkable man and I thank him for and treasure his friendship.

My practice has afforded me and my family a very comfortable living. When I opened the business in 1988, I can recall my mom telling me *to treat every client as if he/she were your only one.* She advised that I not make decisions for the money but because it was the right thing for the client. The money will then come. Again she was right. Not that I am a wealthy person, but I can't complain. Today we still maintain the same level of service and dedication to our clients, and they have stood by me. In that respect, I am rich!

Family, Friends, and Block Island

Thursday, July 17, 2019, was a *very* shitty weather day in Rhode Island. Heavy rain from the remnants of hurricane Barry moved from the Gulf States north to the Mid-Atlantic and then to the northeast part of the country. We were booked for a five day stay at New Harbor Boat Basin on Block Island, Rhode Island, to be with friends for a few days and spend time alone a few more days.

I have always felt it important to keep in touch with family and friends, especially those who were closest to me when I was younger. My friend Peter lived two houses from ours and we became close friends in a very short time. We did everything together and today he is my closest friend. He checks up on me constantly, worries about me driving to and from Boston for treatments and appointments and just cares from the bottom of his heart. We have a very special relationship and most times don't need to speak to know what the other is thinking or feels about something. He is *much* more reserved than I, and he finds that amusing at times.

My sister, Rose, was devastated when I told her of my cancer. She is older than I, and when we were younger, my brother and I thought of her as a grown-up. So we did not tell her things for that reason. Kids will be kids. She is a good person and she calls me often to keep abreast of my progress and how I am doing.

Linda's family has been great too. Her mom, aunts, uncles, and cousins are always keeping in touch. Several of her relatives have offered to drive me to treatments and appointments, worried I am driving alone. I have always refused because this *is my* time, and I get to think about my work, my treatments, and just things in general. It helps me stay focused. Some understand while others don't.

We departed our home port of Wickford Shipyard in Wickford, Rhode Island, about 8:00 a.m. and headed out of Narragansett Bay to the Block Island Sound. Heavy fog as thick as pea soup settled in just south of Point Judith, Rhode Island, and maintained its grip all the way to the island, about twelve miles south. Needless to say, as we approached within five miles of the island, heavy rain from Barry fell. We couldn't see our bow rail as a result of the rain and fog. My radar screen was pure red in color, indicating heavy rain. This meant that other boats in the area, which are normally depicted as red dots on the screen, now appeared as green triangle shapes with the point of the triangle pointed towards the direction of the target's course. This green object certainly helps when you cannot see anything in front or aside of you.

Between Point Judith and the north point of Block Island are shipping lanes where tug boats often pull barges east to Providence, New Bedford, Boston, or west to New York, Connecticut or New Jersey. These barges often carry heavy loads and are connected to the tug boat with thick steel cables that sometimes are a quarter mile long, and due to their length and weight, sag in the middle and are literally under water. Any boat that passes between the tug and the tow is destined for disaster. Should this cable and your propellers meet, chances are your boat will not survive the incident. The cable will win.

In the heavy weather such as we had this day, the tug and tow would most likely not even know this happened, unless the tow boat captain happened to see the approaching vessel on his radar. Often times they travel on auto pilot, though they should not during this type of weather.

Looking at the radar, I could see no such tug and tow operations taking place in front of me. I did see two such operations to the east of us traveling more northwest from the south and about two miles east of me. I knew I was far enough away and past their direction so as not to be in a potential collision situation.

I grew up on boats, and some years ago passed the United States Coast Guard test earning a 100 Ton Master license. I studied and trained with Captain J. Kent Dresser of Confident Captain, in Newport, Rhode Island. I loved studying for that exam and taking the test because during my entire life from childhood, I was running small boats to larger ones when I got old enough. I was a commercial fisherman for many years and always just loved being on the ocean. It seemed to me the testing material not only allowed me to earn a certification for what I loved doing, it reaffirmed my ability to appropriately perform on the water. You see, when running a boat, much comes through instinct. For example, "feeling" the effect of the tide when running a course or docking a boat, comes from experience and first one's instincts. However, when studying for the exam, many test questions addressed how to calculate these tidal effects on one's course through the water, etc. I found this fascinating and so much fun, my wife thought I was somewhat crazy. She would ask, "How could you have so much fun taking a test?"

I would respond that I never felt I was taking a test but just studying what I have been doing my entire life up to now. She would just roll her eyes as if to privately conclude to herself, *He is crazy*!

Heading about two hundred thirty degrees to the 1Bi bouy at the north end of Block Island, I could see the bouy on my radar screen and my GPS Chartplotter. Having approached this green bell numerous times in my life, I knew the target well. But what I saw on the radar screen did not look like how they always did. There were several green triangles circling the bouy. As I approached, I could see with my eyes seven boats with no radar circling the green bouy staying close to it in order to stay out of the shipping lanes and know where they are. The water is about one hundred eighty feet deep, so anchoring there would be a problem for most boats. So they just kept circling the can until the fog and rain subsided. It was a smart thing for them to do. I suppose they could also tie up to the can if they were getting low on fuel, though this should be a last resort.

We approached the breakwater of New Harbor, Block Island, and my wife was very relieved to see land. Once inside the harbor we contacted the New Harbor Boat Basin to let them know we arrived in accordance with our reservation time. We were informed they had no room at the moment because no one would leave due to the weather. Understandable! The marina staff was great, as they were prepared to allow us to temporarily dock at the main pier until the weather cleared a bit, allowing boats scheduled to depart, safe passage. I had no problem with this.

Just as we were preparing for the temporary dockage, the rain stopped and the fog began to lift. Slips began to open up and we were allowed to dock in our reserved slip at the west end of the marina, a *great* place to watch the beautiful Block Island sunsets.

Block Island is and has always been my favorite place on this wonderful Earth. I grew up coming to this island when my dad would take us out fishing and later as a charter captain with me and my brother, Henry, as mates. We had a ball and the island became a second home for us. To me though, it always was a place of solitude and private healing. When I am on Block Island I feel no pain, no stress, no thought of being sick, and have no worries in the world. The fresh salt air allows me to think more clearly and to become one with nature. I don't want to make it seem like I am avoiding reality. I am just saying this place clears the cobwebs of stressful city living from my mind and body, and *that* allows me to face my health issues with more clarity and gives me a sense of reality that I do not experience in the city. I guess you could say being here sort of cleanses my mind and body.

Once we settled in, we were having dinner with some friends and I received an email from my oncologist at Dana-Farber that my test results from Wednesday's visit with Dr. Laubach were ready to view. Excusing myself from the crowd, I opened the e-mail and logged into my portal. What I saw amazed me to the point I thought it was an error. My numbers showed I am in the normal range of the kappa and lambda light chains and the ratio is now in the normal range. Upon reading this, I called to my wife to take a look. She was stunned! I stated to her, "I will hear from him tomorrow if not tonight."

I was referring to Dr. Laubach of course. He always calls me when there is a significant change in my numbers or tests, etc. This is one dedicated professional, and I am blessed to have been able to be his patient. Needless to say, at 4:12 p.m. on July 19, 2019, my cell phone rang and it was Dr. Laubach. "Have you seen your tests from Wednesday, July 17, 2019?" he asked.

"I did," and I asked. "Is it a mistake?"

"No mistake," he said.

We discussed these results and the fact that my immunoglobulins are so low he cannot understand how this is happening so fast. I have only had one full round of treatments, which is four weeks, and one week of the second round. Given my very low immune system, one would think that I would be sick all the time. I very seldom get infections or sick. No one is sure why because as one doctor at Brigham and Women's Hospital told me over ten years ago, "You are the healthiest sick guy I ever met." This was *pre*cancer, but still, the IgG, IgM and IgA readings are so low. Doctors are at a loss to explain why I do not get sick often. The belief is that, this is my base range and somehow my body has a mechanism to counter the job these immunoglobulins should be doing. All I care about is that the body system is working and I seldom get sick. It has been suggested that a study be done to determine what is going on as it may help others with depleted immune systems. I am *all* for it.

When I met with Dr. Laubach on Wednesday, July 17, 2019, at Dana-Farber, we discussed my options. It was pretty much determined that if the chemo was not working this time around, we would not be able to put me in remission. And that is a problem because we had no other options available other than experimental drugs, which have no track record, especially with amyloidosis. However, if the treatments are working, we could do the stem cell replacement.

Stem cell replacement therapy is very interesting. About a year after diagnosis, I submitted to a procedure where an intravenous (IV) access was inserted in each arm. The left IV would take out blood from my body, and the right would replace blood. In the meantime, the extracted blood from my left arm would be put through a machine that would spin the blood and shoot out the stem cells into a bag. I was told by the nurse at the time they would need to extract 8.5 million cells and it usually takes about two to three days. After the first four to five hours on the first day, the nurse came in and stated, "Okay, we are done today."

I then asked what time I should arrive tomorrow and she said, "No, we are done. We have the 8.5 million cells."

I was stunned! "I thought you said it takes two to three days?"

"It usually does," she replied. "But we were able to extract all we need in this short period of time."

I asked her if the machine counted incorrectly and she laughed.

These extracted stem cells will be frozen for up to ten years, during which time they could be infused back into my body if I needed them. These cells would travel throughout and begin the process of killing any other cancer cells. It is an amazing process and one that makes the patient *very* sick for about one week, notwithstanding any infections. It required about two to three weeks hospital admission with a large portion of that in isolation so that there is no exposure to germs, etc. Infections are the main fear in this procedure because the patient's entire immune system is wiped out by heavy doses of chemo prior to the infusion of the stem cells. But there are other risks since the body is going through a complete exchange of cells and blood. The idea is to kill the cancer cells and to replace them with the healthy stem cells taken from my body when I was in remission. Sometimes it works, and other times it doesn't.

My friend Bob had multiple myeloma and was diagnosed one month before I was. He had stem cell replacement therapy but passed away about a year after having it. Yet another friend with the same cancer as Bob had the treatment and is still alive and living a normal life. That's the thing, you invest so much of yourself to the hopes this will work and sometimes it doesn't. It is a last resort of sorts.

In my case, after some discussion of these test results, Dr. Laubach suggested that I now have another option available to me since my body has responded so well and so quickly. He said he would be more than comfortable completing the current rounds of chemo treatments and then administer the maintenance drug as we did the first time I was in remission. Instead of taking me off the maintenance drug, he would keep me on it. He believes this would provide a longer period of remission than the thirteen months I experienced the first time. If the cells begin to become active again, then he would put me back on the treatments, and we could then consider the stem cell therapy. I think he was providing me this option for two reasons:

1. Save the frozen stem cells until we absolutely need them. Last resort!
2. In the time I would be on maintenance, new drugs would emerge that might be available to my situation allowing us to again postpone the last resort. Since I was diagnosed in January 2017, several new drugs have emerged for treating amyloidosis that resulted from the research being done around the world.

I told Dr. Laubach I would take a week to think about this and to discuss with my wife, Linda. I also wanted to discuss it with my other oncologist, Dr. John Reagan, at Rhode Island Hospital. He has been administering the current chemo treatment drugs in accordance with directions from Dana-Farber. This was done so that I would not have to travel to Boston once per week for labs and the next day each week for treatments. Saves time and aggravation from traffic. I have been seeing Dr. Reagan at the request of Dr. Laubach, who works with numerous patients this way. Dr. Reagan and I have had some very frank and helpful discussions, and I trust his judgement. He has been an advocate of the stem cell replacement and expressed so that week when I saw him.

I arrive at Lifespan's East Greenwich, Rhode Island location for my 9:00 a.m. appointment for treatments and to meet with Dr. Reagan to discuss my progress and future plan. Having met with Dr. Laubach at Dana-Farber last Wednesday, we discussed the results of my labs taken there and what Dr. Laubach and I discussed regarding stem cell replacement therapy. Dr. Reagan has been a strong advocate for me having the stem cell replacement therapy. Having had several conversations with him regarding my health and the cancer, he seems to be of the opinion that the best chance of staying off treatments would be to have the stem cell therapy. This was his view prior to my discussions with Dr. Laubach last week.

Stem cell therapy does not extend one's life. It *may* allow for a longer period of time where the cancer patient is not required to have chemo infusions but instead to take maintenance drugs to keep the cells from becoming active again. It does not always work. But when it works, it is nice not to have to take infusions. The drug of choice for maintenance is lenalidamide (Revlimid) Revlimid. This drug is among many that are used in the maintenance area but this is the first choice.

Dr. Reagan and I discussed my status; and I was, in particular, interested in his position regarding the stem cell therapy in light of Dr. Laubach's recent change of opinion to keep me on the maintenance drug instead of the replacement therapy. Being the type of person that I am, I came straight out and asked him, "Have you spoken with Dr. Laubach? And what is your opinion regarding the option to not have the stem cell replacement therapy at this time?"

He responded, "I am comfortable with postponing the stem cell therapy because you responded so well to this treatment."

This was what Dr. Laubach felt as well, and it certainly helped me in making my decision whether to forego the stem cell or not. I decided to postpone this replacement therapy for several reasons:

1. The stem cell therapy will not add additional years of life.
2. With both options, I will need to be on maintenance drugs. The only difference is after stem cell, I will be taking a pill and seeing the doctor every three months. With the remission maintenance, I will need injections every two weeks and see the doctor more often.
3. When the cancer cells begin to become active again, and they will, I will always have the option of stem cell therapy because I have not used the stored cells. These cells are fro-

zen for ten years, and it is widely expected I would relapse in about five years either way.

4. In either case, stem cell or not, I should be in remission for a period of time, perhaps up to five years. During this time, there would be so much more available to me as research is constantly going on and more drugs are being introduced into the marketplace. My position is that during my remission time, it is possible a drug or other treatment will come out that will make stem cell obsolete. Even if I stay on maintenance drugs forever, I am okay with that.

Always Go with Your Gut Feeling

I stated earlier about my initial reluctance to have treatments at Rhode Island Hospital. Having had several treatments at Lifespan's East Greenwich facility, it seemed to me that the administration of the drug used during remission and even in some cases, the full treatment was going quite well. Then it happened. Just as I feared! Things began to unravel with the functions at the facility.

The first time I felt some discomfort with going to Rhode Island Hospital was when I showed for my Velcade shot. The nurse set me up in the chemo room, asked if I needed anything, and then I saw the bag of chemo get delivered. The nurse began setting up the intravenous bag for me when I asked, "What are you doing?"

She said she was getting my treatments set up. I then said that I was there for the Velcade treatment and *not* the full chemotherapy treatments. Well, after about an hour of back-and-forth with Dr. Reagan, they finally agreed that they were about to give me the wrong treatment. Velcade ended up being administered. Someone gave the nurse the wrong order or didn't know what Dr. Laubach wanted done.

The next time things went awry was when I showed up for my appointment around nine one morning. After checking in with the registration person and receiving my wrist band for identification purposes, I sat and worked on this very manuscript for about two hours before someone came out and asked why I was sitting there. When I stated I was waiting for my appointment it was determined that they forgot all about me. It seems that the front desk and the nursing staff did not communicate, and I was just left there. We ended up having the appointment, and things seemed okay for a couple of weeks. Then I was supposed to have a meeting with Dr. Reagan, but he never showed. In my telephone conversation with Dr. Reagan, he stated he was in Providence that day, and someone messed up the schedule. I did receive my Velcade treatment but had to reschedule our meeting for another day.

Finally, the last straw was when I showed up at 9:00 a.m. or so for my treatments, only to be told the medicine was not there! I was stunned and asked the nurse, "What did you say?"

She said the medicine was not delivered and would not arrive for at least two hours. The waiting room was full of people in the same boat. I was stunned and then livid! "I have a business to run," I stated and reiterated my clients' reliance on my ability to meet with them. I had to move appointments at the office because I had to come back for the treatment at 1:00 p.m.

One last comment, when I was, in fact, receiving my Velcade at Rhode Island Hospital, on three weeks in a row, no one asked if I took my Dexamethasone that morning! This steroid is critical in the Velcade treatments. I never said anything to anyone because I knew I took it.

Needless to say, I phoned Dr. Laubach at Dana-Farber and told him of the events. His response was, "Get back up here!"

So I cancelled all scheduled appointments at Rhode Island Hospital and again began my Velcade treatments at Dana-Farber. My story is one that proves that your initial gut feelings are the ones you should follow when dealing with cancer or any other disease. Do not make alterations to your treatment schedule or any other aspects of your treatments just for the sake of convenience. I thought that going to Rhode Island Hospital for a simple injection every two weeks would be a simple thing, and that nothing could go wrong. Boy, was I wrong! Follow the best course of action and with the best facility regardless of the inconvenience it may impose. Your life depends on it!

Amyloidosis

I mentioned that the type of cancer I have is multiple myeloma and amyloidosis. The former is somewhat common these days and is treated with certain chemo and other drugs. No cure for this cancer, but people can live long lives if caught early and treated properly. My readings have been so low it appears the multiple myeloma is no longer measurable. *Amazing!*

Amyloidosis is another story. Very rare and incurable at this time, it is somewhat a silent killer. You see once a person develops symptoms of this cancer, it is probably too late to help. I was not having any symptoms except in August of 2016. I complained to a local doctor of shortness of breath when I walked up a short flight of stairs at the office. He examined me and said my asthma was back and prescribed an inhaler. So after using the inhaler for a short time I cannot say there was any difference. Then I attended my appointment with Dr. Emily Robinson at Brigham and Women's Hospital. *Bingo!* No asthma, *cancer!* I find it amazing that a doctor could be so wrong and not know it. I complained to him later to no avail. This was evidence to me that some doctors, as with any profession, don't know what they don't know. *Very scary!*

The point here is that each of us cannot just rely on what a single doctor says. They express *opinions,* and we all know that opinions are like assholes, everyone has one. Dr. Robinson was very quick to determine there was and still is no asthma. The cancer hit my heart and kidneys, and the result was shortness of breath. This cancer has permanently impacted these organs. However, we learn to cope, and in my case, I found different ways of breathing when I exert myself. The only long-term effect I still cannot seem to learn to adjust to, but I will, is when I bend over or kneel and lean forward, I lose my breath. So I try to avoid these positions as much as I can. Again I learned to find a way to adjust to the new "me."

Actual root causes of amyloidosis are sometimes offered, but the truth is no one really knows. Research is being done at rapid paces, and I feel comfortable they will nail it down soon. Symptoms of this cancer are shown below according to the Amyloidosis foundation.[1] The thing to remember is it really doesn't matter to me *how* I ended up with this cancer because there isn't anything I can do to change that. It happened, and I need to deal with it. If I spend time trying to figure out what *could* have caused it, I would never find time to live. I will be thinking all day and night, to no avail and with no positive results or gain from this. Look forward, not back, and it will help you learn about your body as it is *now* and not what could have been or what might have changed had I not done this or that. Water under the bridge at this point.

---

[1] www.amyloidosis.org

A few symptoms of Amyloidosis:

What is AL Amyloidosis?

AL amyloidosis is caused by a bone marrow disorder. Misfolded proteins can accumulate in the body's tissue, nerves and/or organs, gradually causing damage and affecting function.

amyloidosis foundation

Symptoms may include:

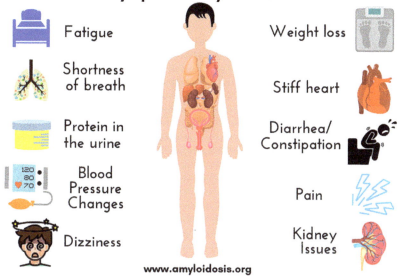

Fatigue

Shortness of breath

Protein in the urine

Blood Pressure Changes

Dizziness

Weight loss

Stiff heart

Diarrhea/ Constipation

Pain

Kidney Issues

www.amyloidosis.org

The only symptom I had besides the shortness of breath was the protein in the urine. As stated earlier, that is what alerted Dr. Robinson to investigate further. Thanks to her, this cancer was caught early and treatments have been relatively successful.

According to the Amyloidosis Foundation:

> Amyloidosis is caused by changes in proteins that make them insoluble, leading them to deposit in organs and tissues. These amyloid proteins accumulate mainly in the tissue space between cells.

Changes in proteins that make them amyloid proteins occur because of gene mutations.[2]

Again research needs to be done to determine what causes these gene mutations to occur.

Amyloidosis (am-uh-loi-DO-sis) is a rare disease that occurs when a substance called amyloid builds up in your organs. Amyloid is an abnormal protein that is produced in your bone marrow and can be deposited in any tissue or organ. Amyloidosis can affect different organs in different people, and there are different types of amyloid. Amyloidosis frequently affects the heart, kidneys, liver, spleen, nervous system and digestive tract. Severe amyloidosis can lead to life-threatening organ failure. There's no cure for amyloidosis. But treatments can help you manage your symptoms and limit the production of amyloid protein.[3] Amyloidosis is often overlooked because the signs and symptoms can mimic those of more common diseases.

In my case, I was short of breath a bit and only at times. Diagnosis as early as possible can help prevent further organ damage. Precise diagnosis is important because treatment varies greatly, depending on your specific condition.[4]

In my case, these proteins impacted my heart, kidneys, and bone marrow where they originate.

My understanding is that these proteins will get into the walls of the organs and "thicken" them. It reminds me of barnacles gather-

---

[2]   www.amyloidosis.org

[3]   https://www.mayoclinic.org/diseases-conditions/amyloidosis/diagnosis-treatment/drc-20353183

[4]   https://www.mayoclinic.org/diseases-conditions/amyloidosis/diagnosis-treatment/drc-20353183

ing on an underwater object. They latch onto the item and thicken its length and width. When these deposits get too far and untreated, the walls of the organ can thicken to the point that the patient has symptoms. If not caught early, the organ can literally suffocate.

An otherwise healthy person would not notice any shortness of breath unless he/she is very much "in tune" with his/her own body. This was what happened in my case. Generally very healthy and active, I only noticed a limited shortness of breath and questioned it. If I was not "in tune" with my body the way I am, I probably would never have noticed until it was more advanced.

Teaching moment—listen to your body and be aware of small changes. Always follow up on these changes. They may be nothing, or they may be something critical.

Critical Test Results

One day before each treatment, I have blood drawn so that the oncologist and nurses can determine if my kidneys are functioning properly. If they are not, then I cannot take the chemo. However, on the first of each month, a more extensive blood test is required in order to determine if the chemo is working. This is a big deal and requires the measurement of the lambda light chain cells in my body. These light chain cells are the cancer cells that are all the trouble. Another measurement is the kappa cells. The ratio of kappa to lambda is a critical measurement as well. This tells the team whether the chemo is doing its job. The three numbers must fall between a high and a low. If these numbers fall outside the range, then the drugs are not working, and trouble begins.

One day, I was at Rhode Island Hospital for my labs and the next day my chemo infusion. The kappa, lambda, and ratio from the labs were not encouraging. Dr. Reagan and I sat down during my chemo infusion and discussed the results. Both he and I were somewhat disappointed with these numbers. We discussed the next steps according to his opinion, and the topic of stem cell replacement therapy came up again. He also mentioned the possibility of increasing the steroid (Dexamethasone) that I am taking on the day of chemo infusion. This steroid sort of stimulates the chemo and makes it more effective. I am on a lower dose of the steroid because it makes my heart beat considerably faster with the higher the dose.

At the current level, the heart beats at about 90 bpm rather than 150 bpm on the higher dose.

Needless to say, I was somewhat disappointed by the test results and our discussions. So I called Dr. Laubach at Dana-Farber and asked him to look at the results. He immediately ordered the same blood labs to be taken at Dana-Farber on the Friday afternoon. So I went to Boston and had the labs done.

It was Labor Day weekend 2019, so on Friday evening, Dr. Laubach called me and said the results would probably not be back until after Labor Day. Normally these labs come back within twenty-four hours. I understood this and spent the weekend doing jobs around the yard and the boat. I did not think much about what the labs showed at Rhode Island Hospital because I really do not use them as the actual results; more of a guide. The results from Dana-Farber would be gospel to me. So, Linda and I spent the weekend doing things we love doing.

On Tuesday morning I received the results and was astonished! These labs showed a 20 percent decrease in the lambda light chain cells, while the results of Rhode Island Hospital showed a 0.4 point decrease *and* the lambda level was 50 percent lower from Dana-Farber than that measured by Rhode Island Hospital. Unbelievable!

Today, which is Wednesday, September 4, 2019, Dr. Laubach called my cell phone, just as I told my wife, Linda, he would. He was very encouraged by the results, and we discussed the plan that we discussed previously: stem cell therapy versus continued chemo maintenance.

One might wonder how a blood test from one lab could be so different from that of another lab. I am told that each lab performs the test differently and with a different assay. While I understand this as a possible cause for different measured results, when the spread is 50 percent, *that* is *huge!* One test tells the doctors that the chemo is not working while the other tells them that I am responding very well to the chemo. Below are my numbers from Rhode Island Hospital and those from Dana-Farber for July17, 2019 and August 30, 2019:

	Rhode Island Hospital			Dana-Farber		
			Percent			Percent
	July	Aug	Change	July	Aug	Change
Kappa Light Chain	7.8	7.9	1.28	6.7	6.6	1.49
Lambda Light Chain	35.2	34.8	(1.14)	22	17.6	(20.00)
Ratio	0.22	0.23	4.55	0.3	0.38	26.67

Looking at these numbers, one can see the difference in results from Rhode Island Hospital and Dana-Farber for the same lab tests. Rhode Island Hospital showed a 1.28 percent increase in kappa light chains while Dana-Farber showed a 1.49 percent increase. But look at the levels from each. They are about 1.3 points lower at Dana-Farber.

The critical number lambda light chain shows a decrease of 1.14 percent at Rhode Island Hospital while Dana-Farber shows a decrease of 20 percent. Again look at the levels. In August 2019, Rhode Island Hospital had my lambda light chains at 34.8 while Dana-Farber had them at 17.6. This is an astounding 49.4 percent difference. Almost 50 percent difference in the level of these cells. In essence, Dana-Farber has me in remission again while Rhode Island Hospital has me showing a slower response to the chemo and *not* in remission. You will note that this occurred two months in a row, July and August.

Let's take a look at the ratio. Rhode Island Hospital showed a ratio of 0.22 and 0.23, a 4.5 percent increase in July and August, respectively, while Dana-Farber showed a ratio of 0.30 and 0.38, or a 26.6 percent increase. These differences are enormous when talking about cancer cells. Again, one set of numbers shows me slowing in response to the chemo (Rhode Island Hospital) while another shows a significant response and improvement (Dana-Farber) and indicates for a second month that I am in remission.

Dr. Laubach and I spoke about this and what we do next. He was not even considering the lab results from Rhode Island Hospital because he relies solely on the Dana-Farber results. I do too. Not because they are better in these above tests but because Dana-Farber is *the* cancer institute in the country, and I have all the confidence in the world in their people and practices. The lab technicians at Dana-Farber test for *cancer* and nothing else. No TB, hepatitis, or other disorders. Just cancer! This is their thing, and I believe it makes all the difference in the world. This is why I initially decided to have treatments at Dana-Farber and not Rhode Island Hospital for my initial therapy. I still stand by this, and while the long drive is some-what burdensome, it is a small price to pay for the best in the country and possibly the world.

Please do not take my opinion in the wrong context. My experience with the nurses and doctors at Rhode Island Hospital was very good. However, the people at Dana-Farber see so much more, participate in so much research and trials, etc., that one cannot compare the two. I mentioned earlier in a previous chapter the fact that I was participating in research studies. Well this afforded me access to treatment and tests and information that my doctors could use to help treat me and extend my life. I doubt Rhode Island Hospital could or would have done this right from the outset as Dana-Farber did. *It makes a huge difference!*

As a result of these differences two months in a row, Dr. Laubach and I agreed that I would have the test performed at Dana-Farber the same time Rhode Island Hospital performs it each month. I will travel to Boston to have this done. However, Dana-Farber is scheduled to open a facility in Foxboro, Massachusetts, at Patriot Place. This is the development where the New England Patriots have their home stadium, Gillette Stadium. This is about the same distance from my house and office as Rhode Island Hospital's East Greenwich location. So that will be great. I can go there for labs and infusion each week. The only mistake I made here is the initial reading of the light chains by Rhode Island Hospital at fifty-one, which should have been followed up at Dana-Farber. I never thought of it because at the time, it never occurred to me that the readings would be so different. Looking at the variances of the two months, I wonder if the results would have suggested I was still in remission and did not need the second series of infusions being administered. We will never know.

The key here is that, as patients, we think a blood test is a blood test. I have come to learn that this is not the case. Each lab performs the analysis differently, and this makes the end result different. After my initial episode, I spoke with several people in the medical field, mostly nurses, and they all agreed that it all depends on which lab the patient goes to. Frightening!

Another key lab test that is determined from my blood is my creatinine level. Creatinine is a measure of the function of the kidneys. If this level is not within a certain range, administration of the chemotherapy is not an option. In order to administer the chemo, the kidneys must be functioning properly.

Having had such a variance in the results of the light chains from Rhode Island Hospital and Dana-Farber, I decided to schedule out the creatinine levels taken at Rhode Island hospital and compare them to my readings from Dana-Farber. The results are depicted below.

	Rhode Island Hospital		Dana-Farber	
	July	August	July	August
Creatinine	1.33	1.45	1.34	1.56

Looking at the chart of the results, we can see that although the numbers move up and down each day, they are fairly consistent between the two organizations. Creatinine levels will fluctuate daily depending on several factors. One such factor is if the patient has not been drinking enough water. This will significantly alter the levels of creatinine. Another is if there is an infection in the body that is not known. For example, I have found that if I have had a reaction to food that I ate, my creatinine levels will fluctuate. The good thing is that the results from each institution shows a trend of a properly functioning kidney. As I write this passage, my creatinine levels read 1.15. Thank God because the last thing I want is to have kidneys that are not working properly to mess things up even further.

Oh Boy—Another Cancer

So it turns out that in August 2018 I had a slightly elevated PSA count. Dr. Martin Kathrins of Brigham and Women's Hospital recommended a biopsy of the prostate as a precaution given the situation with the other cancers I have, and then, if positive, an MRI to determine the scope of the prostate cancer.

We immediately took twelve biopsy samples from the gland and two from the left side of the prostate were cancerous. Given this result, Dr. Kathrins ordered an MRI to measure more accurately the scope of the cancer and whether it spread beyond the gland. The result was that it is contained within the two sections that the biopsy suggested and, thankfully, had not gone beyond the prostate gland.

Next step was to consult a qualified prostate doctor considering not only the prostate cancer *but* the impact of treatment and other matters given my other cancers. Dr. Kathrins recommended a doctor from Brigham and Women's, and I asked him if he knew a Dr. Anthony D'Amico from Dana-Farber. He was not familiar with this doctor so I decided to consult my Oncologist at Dana-Farber, Jacob Laubach, who knew of him and all Dr. D'Amico is known for. He stated he has an outstanding reputation and success rate and he would have no problem recommending and working with him.

I found out about Dr. D'Amico by accident. About two years before I was diagnosed with prostate cancer, a very close friend of my father told me of his diagnosis of prostate cancer. He stated that after meeting with his doctor in Rhode Island and other doctors who treat this disease, he was frustrated and expressed his concerns to his primary care doctor. The concerns were principally that the doctors in Rhode Island wanted to cut him open and remove the gland and other things he was not comfortable with. After expressing his concerns, he told me his doctor heard about Dr. D'Amico in Boston at Dana-Farber and that he is working wonders with new treatments and not surgery. So of course, he pursued the matter and found that was exactly the case. Dad's friend told me that if I ever needed treatment for this type of cancer to look up Dr. D'Amico. So I did.

My wife and I met with Dr. D'Amico in September 2019 and he spent a considerable amount of time explaining the various treatments, effects of each treatment and then recommended what treatment he was comfortable providing me. Of concern in all of his studying my case was and still is the impact of the chemo drugs I have been on for the multiple myeloma and amyloidosis and various steroids etc. While I was concerned with this as well, it was out of my pay grade to make the determination, at least at that time. So after Dr. D'Amico and I discussed the ultimate effects of each on my body, we agreed to implant radioactive pellets and radiate the gland over a five-day period. His prognosis was that he would be able to eradicate the prostate cancer with 99.9 percent surety. I was delighted, as was my wife.

A few months went by, and I started to get a little concerned that I was not hearing from anyone to set up the meetings and visits necessary to educate me and get the matter moving. You see, Dr. D'Amico indicated that in order to prepare my body for the radiation treatments, I must be off chemo. It was the end of October 2019, and I had not heard from anyone, so I got the ball rolling. I called Dr. D'Amico's office and my oncologist, Dr. Laubach. My discussions with Dr. Laubach were *very* productive as usual, and he inserted me into his schedule for the next week to discuss this matter further and in person. Shortly after my telephone discussion with Dr.

Laubach, I heard from Dr. D'Amico. We discussed the plan, and it seems he is concerned that too heavy doses of radiation would have a detrimental impact on my kidneys, bladder, and possibly rectum. So he decided we would administer the radiation every day for nine weeks *after* I receive hormone therapy for four months. Yikes!

My concern was that we needed to get me beyond tax-filing season because I service, with my staff, hundreds of clients during the months of January through April 15. Dr. D'Amico and Dr. Laubach therefore scheduled things to work around this hectic time. The nine weeks of radiation will start shortly after April 15. This works out *great*!

So on November 13, 2019, I met with two more oncologists. One is a medical oncologist to discuss the approach and pros and cons to the treatment. He asked if I spoke with a surgeon regarding the prostate cancer, to which I replied no.

He suggested I speak with an oncology surgeon to be aware of all the options. Within one hour, I was sitting with Chief of Prostate Surgery, and we discussed the surgical aspects of the treatments. Several topics were discussed, including, but not limited to, the short- and long-term effects of surgery. Basically, it comes down to this: Surgery will leave me incontinent for the rest of my life, *but* there would be no chance of additional cancer in *that* specific organ because the organ is *gone*! There are remedies to the incontinence that included either some device being inserted into the urethra or a pump device that would have a valve on it that would have to be opened each time I needed to urinate. This conversation did *not* give me any good feelings.

One reason the medical oncologist wanted me to hear the surgery option is because, radiation *can* cause other cancer. For example, it could cause bladder or rectal cancer. The odds are quite low, about 1–3 percent according to the medical oncologist. But still there nonetheless.

I made all my notes regarding my discussions with both the medical and surgical oncologists and then made a call to Dr. Anthony D'Amico, who called me back within one hour. I mentioned the surgery option to him and asked to refresh my memory on the odds that the radiation would cause another cancer. He stated, as he did to my initial inquiry at our first meeting, less than 1 percent, in fact he stated one in three hundred chance. Further, the onset would take ten to fifteen years.

I mentioned to Dr. D'Amico my concerns, and within a few minutes, I felt much better about the radiation treatment. But I then received a call from Dr. Laubach, who saw I was active at the hospital that day. We discussed my meetings with the surgeon and medical oncologist and my discussion with Dr. D'Amico. Dr. Laubach was very helpful, and when I asked him what he thought was the better way for me to go, he stated radiation with *no* hesitation. That was all it took to cement my own feelings, but I think I just needed to hear it from someone who was knowledgeable about the topic and whom I trusted with my life. That person is Jacob Laubach. The decision is made, and we proceeded as planned.

On June 30, 2020, I began the process of executing the plan to eradicate the prostate cancer by attending a "planning" session at the Radiation Oncology Department. On this day, I was scheduled for and received a CT scan of the pelvic area and was given my first ever tattoo. Three *very* small marks were made on my pelvic area marking the site where the radiation needs to be aimed. These marks depicted the area determined by triangulation resulting from the MRI and CT scan I received. Pointing the radiation to these marks would pinpoint the site of the gold markers inserted in me weeks ago and attempting to "zap" the cancer cells over a period of sixty-two days, forty-four treatments. Having been on chemo for the last three and one-half years makes my internal organs and veins more susceptible to damage should the radiation be too strong. Therefore, Dr. D'Amico decided to administer the "dosage" of each treatment at a lower level than normal but over an extended period of time. This poses an inconvenience of having to drive to Boston for the forty-four days, *but* a small price to pay versus the alternative risks.

My Saviors

I wanted to offer some attention to the team of doctors who have been and continue to be so much a part of my life and who have kept me alive. These are not just doctors working in their professions. They are compassionate and dedicated people who make their field of study their lives. They are pioneers in their area of expertise, and they certainly are the people who have kept me alive to this day.

There are so many others I could mention, but I do not know all of their names. These are the nurses and technicians at both Dana-Farber, Brigham and Women's, and Rhode Island Hospital. My main nurse at Dana-Farber was without a doubt the most dedicated and professional nurse I have ever met or worked with. These people are the real deal, and they care immensely for those they treat. It is truly a pleasure to see them every week, notwithstanding the reason I am there.

One of the most notable people I met at Dana-Farber is nurse practitioner to Dr. Jacob Laubach. This woman is a no-bullshit person and cares for her patients from the bottom to the top of her heart and with every single bone in her body. Some people don't like her approach because she tells it like it is. But I recognized early on that she is dedicated, cares about doing the best she can at her profession, and will help a patient with *anything* she can at any time. I cherish this wonderful person and consider her a true friend. Her name is not published here because she does not like to take center stage. She prefers to work in the background. I respect that.

I included photos of the doctors I mentioned here. These are the captains of the ship that is being steered, and the nurses and technicians are the engine, sails, and other functioning aspects of the ship. Without the knowledge and dedication of these doctors, I would not be alive today. Perhaps this cancer will eventually end my life, but for now these are the people keeping me alive and living a normal life. They are truly special people who will have a special spot in heaven.

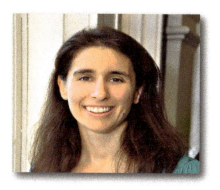

Dr. Emily Robinson, Nephrologist, Brigham and Women's Hospital in Boston

Medical School
    University of Connecticut School of Medicine

Board Certifications
    Internal Medicine, 2006
    Nephrology, 2008

Fellowship
    Brigham and Women's/Massachusetts General Joint Nephrology Fellowship, 2006–2009[5]

---

[5] www.brighamandwomens.org

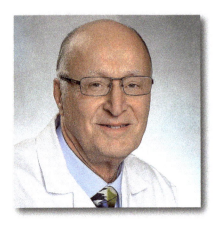

Dr. Rodney Falk, Cardiologist, Brigham and Women's Hospital, Boston, Massachusetts

Medical School
    University of Birmingham Medical School

Residencies
    Brook General Hospital, 1976–1977
    Kings College Hospital, 1977–1978

Board Certifications
    Internal Medicine, 1980
    Cardiovascular Disease, 1981

Fellowship
    Harvard School of Public Health, 1978–1980

Dr. Rodney H. Falk is the director of the Cardiac Amyloidosis Program and a cardiovascular medicine specialist at Brigham and Women's Hospital (BWH). He is also an associate professor of medicine at Harvard Medical School.

Dr. Falk received his medical degree from the University of Birmingham Medical School in the United Kingdom. He then completed three residencies: an internal medicine program at Brook

General Hospital, an internal medicine program at City Hospital and a cardiology program at King's College Hospital—all in London. He also completed a cardiology fellowship at Harvard School of Public Health. Dr. Falk is board certified in internal medicine and cardio-vascular disease. The author of over one hundred peer-reviewed publications, Dr. Falk's research focuses on understanding cardiac amyloidosis and treatment of this rare disease. His research has been supported by the National Institutes of Health.

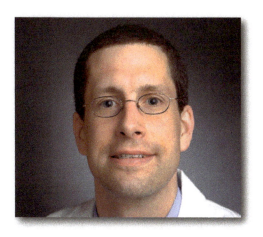

Dr. Jacob Laubach, Oncologist, Dana-Farber Cancer Institute

Board Certification:
    Hematology, 2009
    Internal Medicine, 2012
    Medical Oncology, 2008

Fellowship:
    Duke University School of Medicine, Hematology Oncology

Residency:
    Duke University School of Medicine, Internal Medicine

Medical School:
Duke University School of Medicine

Dr. Laubach received his medical degree from Duke University School of Medicine in 1999. He completed his residency in internal medicine and his fellowship in hematology oncology at the same school. He received board certification from the American Board of Internal Medicine in 2002 and from the American Board of Medical Oncology in 2008.

In 2008, he joined the staff of Dana-Farber and Brigham and Women's Hospital, where he is a medical oncologist and clinical investigator in the Hematologic Malignancies Center, focusing on multiple myeloma as an area of expertise.[6]

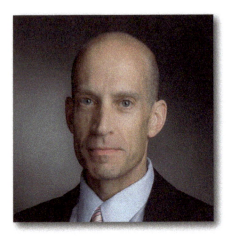

Dr. Anthony D'Amico, Oncologist at Dana-Farber Cancer Institute

Dr. Anthony D'Amico is the Eleanor Theresa Walters distinguished Chair, Chief of Genitourinary Radiation Oncology at the Dana-Farber Cancer Institute and Brigham and Women's Hospital, Chair of the residency executive committee in the Harvard Radiation

---

[6] www.dana-farber.org

Oncology Program, and Advisory Dean and Chair of career advising and mentorship at Harvard Medical School.

Dr. D'Amico is an internationally known expert in the treatment of prostate cancer and has defined combined modality staging, which is used to select patients with localized prostate cancer for specific surgical or radiotherapeutic treatment options. He is the principal investigator of several federally funded grants that support his investigations in Image Guided Therapy for early-stage prostate cancer, drug development for advanced-stage prostate cancer, and clinical trials that are aimed at defining future management strategies for men with prostate cancer.

Dr. Anthony D'Amico is currently developing and testing molecular imaging in addition to collaborating in identifying genomic risk classification profiles, which hold promise for significantly improving the way in which prostate cancer is detected and treated leading us to personalization of prostate cancer care

Dr. D'Amico holds two undergraduate and three graduate degrees: a BS in physics, a BS in nuclear engineering, MS in nuclear engineering, and a PhD in radiation physics, all from the Massachusetts Institute of Technology, and an MD from the University of Pennsylvania School of Medicine. He completed his residency in the Department of Radiation Oncology of the Hospital of the University of Pennsylvania in Philadelphia, where he served as chief resident during his final year. He has over 350 peer-reviewed original publications and editorials, and his teaching contributions include his position as head of the executive committee of the Harvard Combined Residency in Radiation Oncology, Master of the Oliver Wendell Holmes Society at Harvard Medical School, editorial board member of six scientific journals, expert reviewer for fourteen journals including the *New England Journal of Medicine* and the *Journal of the American Medical Association* and editor of four textbooks on the management of prostate cancer.

Dr. D'Amico has been awarded the Best Doctor in America Award annually since 2009 for his work in prostate cancer; the 2012 Harvard Medical School Arnold P. Gold Awardee for Humanism in Medicine; the HMS Faculty Mentoring and Teaching Award in

2014, 2015 and 2017; and the recipient of the Harvard Medical School Class of 2014, 2015 Career Advising and Mentoring Faculty Teaching Award in addition to the 2015–2016 Morton M. Kligerman Award provided by the Hospital of the University of Pennsylvania. In December of 2016, his editorial on a landmark prostate cancer study in the *New England Journal of Medicine* was cited in *The New Yorker* as one of the most notable medical findings in 2016. In 2019, he was awarded the Grant V. Rodkey, MD Award for Outstanding Contributions to Medical Education.

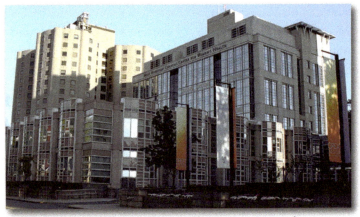

Brigham and Women's Hospital, Boston, Massachusetts

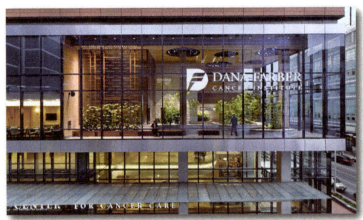

Dana–Farber Cancer institute, Boston, Massachusetts

Remission

On Wednesday, November 20, 2019, I was given a chemo treatment for the multiple myeloma and amyloidosis, and I was supposed to have my last treatment on Wednesday before Thanksgiving. I called Dr. Laubach and asked if we could move this treatment to Monday before Thanksgiving because usually the day after treatment is a difficult day for me, and I probably would not participate in the holiday activities. He responded that we could actually skip the last treatment and start on the maintenance drug Velcade but that I still would need to take the steroids. I was on board with this as long as he was confident it would not impact my progress. He was *very* confident.

So we started the maintenance drug and steroids on the Friday after Thanksgiving. Everything went well, and the schedule was for me to have this type of treatment every two weeks until further notice. I believe the plan is to stop these treatments about a week before the radiation and then resume after the radiation. No sweat with me!

With the news of being in remission again, I asked Dr. Laubach if I could fly on a commercial airplane. He said as long as I wear a mask, use plenty of hand sanitizer, and wipe everything with which I come in contact with bleach wipes.

COVID-19

On December 4, 2019, I was riding on a train from Providence to Boston and should arrive in an hour or so. This trip was to have labs drawn at Dana-Farber and to meet with the scheduler for the prostate hormone therapy and radiation etc. This is good because it provides plenty of time for me to plan around the tests and other events related to the prostate treatments. My goal is to schedule out the entire process on this day so that we can get through this issue with minimal delay or setbacks. I arrived at the Back Bay in Boston, then called an Uber for the trip to Dana-Farber. The reverse to return.

Everything went very well, so we scheduled to have "markers" installed in my prostate where the radiation would be focused come April 2020. The procedure for inserting was uncomfortable, but not the worst thing I've been through. It took about ten minutes, and off I went back to the office.

We were scheduled to begin radiation April 20, 2020, and I was to be taken off Velcade chemo at least a week before the radiation started. We would resume after radiation was complete. All things going well, Linda and I decided to fly to Naples, Florida, for a few days to catch some sunshine and enjoy some time together. It has been a hectic three years. So in December, we took a trip to Naples and fell in love with the place. Driving throughout the entire town, we found several areas we loved, one being the Gulf Coast, of course, but also downtown Naples. This is *the* place! We spent time in the downtown area and really loved the town.

We met a young man at the resort whose job was valet parking. He was from Rhode Island and actually lived one street from my wife's parents. Getting to know Cory a bit and expressing our interest in buying a house in Naples, he provided us with a realtor's name and number.

Our realtor is from the Midwest and relocated to Naples after working in the fashion industry for some years. He showed us around the area of Naples and took us to several properties. When we returned to Rhode Island, he continued to provide leads on property every day. Then it happened! He phoned me and stated that a developer purchased an entire block just outside downtown Naples and is building a gated community. We took a flight a few days later to meet with the sales representative and look at the location. *Perfect!* After some negotiations and documentation, we sent a deposit and signed papers to build a new home in this gated community.

All excited, my wife and I began planning our next trip down to pick out cabinets, counter tops, flooring, etc. Nope! COVID-19 arrived in the United States, and there was no way I was flying. It was tax season so I could not drive. Even if I could, where would we stay? Hotels are public places, and we would not know the virus was not in the hotel! Additionally, I needed to be in Boston for my treatments every other week. Time was an issue as was the virus. So now we had to wait out the virus.

After lockdowns in Rhode Island and many other states, we decided to rent a camper and drive to Florida. I rented a twenty-five-foot camper, had the cleaning team I use for my office sterilize the entire inside with hospital sterilization products, and we packed up the camper and headed out for Naples.

About two weeks before we left for Naples, I purchased a convertible Ford Mustang from a dealer in Fort Myers, Florida. The agreement was that if we did not like the car when we saw it, we could apply the money we paid towards the purchase of another vehicle.

We arrived in Fort Myers on June 16, 2020, and went straight to the dealership. The camper was covered in bugs splattered over the entire front and windshield of the vehicle. I saw a man in the lot and asked if I could get someone to wash the camper for me. After I identified myself, he knew we purchased a car there and said he would wash it for me. I slipped him $50, and for the next hour, he washed every inch of that camper. We were amazed how much effort and time this man put into cleaning the bugs off that vehicle. Turns out he is the dealership manager! I would have thought he would call one of the yard hands to clean it, but he did it himself. Amazing!

The manager called one of his employees and had our car brought out for us to see. We loved it. Now, my wife drove the car, and I dove the camper to the Public Storage at 3232 Colonial Blvd in Fort Myers, Florida. They stored the camper outside for less than $30 *for a month*! Unbelievable! We only needed about ten or twelve days, but if we did need to stay longer, no problem.

Radiation Planning

I n late March early April 2020, I had a telephone discussion with Dr. Laubach about coming to Boston for treatments. COVID-19 resulted in a delay of the continuation of treatments, so he and I decided that it would be best to postpone the current treatment and wait to see what happens for two more weeks. We resumed the treatments, and on July 5, 2020, I received my last chemo treatment before I begin radiation treatments for the prostate cancer.

The week before the actual radiation treatment, I attended the radiation planning session on level 2 at Brigham and Women's Hospital. There I was given a CT scan and MRI to determine the exact location of my prostate at this time. I guess it is possible that the prostate moved around over time, and the doctor wanted to be certain he was to aim the radiation exactly where it needed to be aimed. I was all for this because I certainly would not want the treatments to miss the area with the cancer. When they took the biopsy several months ago, it was determined that I had two areas on the left side of my prostate that were cancerous. Other areas of the prostate where they took samples apparently came back okay. So I am grateful they performed these scans to find the exact location of the cancer.

I have always believed that everything a person does creates a wake, similar to that produced by the movement of a boat through the water that affects others. I further believe that we all need to be cognizant of this wake so that we are careful not to impact others in a negative way.

I experienced something that stunned me. After my radiation planning session, I was waiting for the elevator at level 2 at Brigham and Women's Hospital. A woman was waiting for an elevator going up as I was. When the car arrived, there was another woman already in the car, and so we proceeded to enter. Note that there are signs next to the elevator buttons on each floor stating, "Maximum of 4 people due to COVID-19." Since there were only three of us on the elevator, we were okay. The car stopped at level 1, and five doctors entered the car. That would make eight people in this car—twice the allowed number of passengers according to the current policy. Immediately I exited the car at level 1 and waited for another car to arrive to bring me to my destination, floor 3.

Imagine, *doctors* not adhering to the policy set forth to protect patients and others from contracting COVID. Needless to say, I was pissed off. So when I was driving home, I called patient relations at Brigham and Women's and told of my experience. This person was mortified and promised to look into the matter. I then called my prostate oncologist, Dr. D'Amico, and he too was mortified. I explained that I would be writing a letter to the president of the hospital because if the chief doesn't know what the others are doing, policy cannot be properly instituted. Accordingly, I wrote to Dr. Betsy Nable, president of Brigham and Women's Hospital, and outlined my experience.

The next weekend, I was visiting a friend on his boat and ran into someone who works at the Brigham and Women's Hospital. I mentioned my experience and immediately the person exclaimed, "That was *you?*"

I said *yes* and told my entire experience. The individual mentioned that every worker and department head received a letter from the president of the hospital and also the matter hit the hospital's newsletter. I was provided a copy of the newsletter and was glad to find out something was being done.

The following Monday, I had my daily radiation appointment and decided to wait at the main floor elevators to see how many marked dots were on the floor of the car indicating to passengers where to stand. I counted seven marks. Now these marks are not two feet apart, so it appears the policy itself is flawed. I also noticed the signs that I saw last week at the elevator doors indicating maximum of four people were removed. My only conclusion is that the president notified the department heads who reprimanded the staff and then removed the safety precautions initially instituted at the hospital so as not to be out of compliance with policy. In other words, they changed the policy to a less protective one instead of enforcing the original policy to protect the hospital workers as well as the patients they are supposed to care for. Unbelievable!

We all know that water flows downstream, and if the water from up above is dirty, then the dirt is carried with the flow. In this case, someone in upper management of the hospital did not care enough to enforce safe policy but opted to reduce the inconvenience of strict policy aimed at saving lives.

On July 21, 2020, I had my fifth radiation treatment. I did not experience any issues because I was taking the D elevators, which are reserved for staff only. But today I was on the L and M elevators as the staff was using the D cars. Here is what happened: On the L elevators, I was riding with one other woman when four people dressed in "blues" attempted to enter the car. I immediately stopped after two of them entered the car. The others were to wait for another elevator. When I did this, I cited, "How can we possibly stay six feet apart?"

They did not enter the car but looked at me as if I was a crazy man. The next episode was actually on the main M elevators. Two people with caps on (they looked like they worked in laundry) were wheeling two large baskets. One entered the elevator while the other started to enter. I asserted she wait for the next car. She grunted at me! Imagine that! A patient trying to stay safe is being grunted at by hospital employees because they are inconvenienced in keeping with CDC guidelines.

After all of this, I walked over to 15 Francis Street where President Nagel's office is. When I asked the guard where her office is, he would not tell me. So I attempted to call her and was screened and told I needed to call patient relations. It was like they were protecting the president of the hospital from pain-in-the-ass patients.

Utterly frustrated, I then walked over to patient relations at 75 Francis Street only to find out my contact there is working from home today. However, within half hour, she called me, and I explained the events of the day. She was more upset than I because *she* attended the meetings with the hospital department heads to discuss this matter, and it is still happening. My last straw is to write another letter to the president outlining the current status and the incidents I ran into that day.

I wrote a second letter to President Nagle and outlined the events that occurred subsequent to my first letter. *Now* I saw a difference after about three days. No longer are there so many people getting on the elevator cars. They are waiting for another car. This is what is supposed to happen. However, these people are supposed to know this and practice it without having to be scolded like delinquent children. The good news is, the problem is solved!

Always Try to Move Forward

Despite the issues mentioned above, I always keep in mind the need to constantly move forward. I cannot allow other people's lack of consideration and respect for others, or their selfish behavior, to have any impact on my mission, which is to constantly move forward with the goal of eradicating all the cancer in my body. No one else is going to do this for me. Therefore, it is imperative to maintain a positive attitude and to always keep the goal in my sights. To do anything else is, in my mind, weakness and *that* will eventually lead to defeat. Remember, the cancer is trying as hard as it can to kill me. Therefore, if I let my guard down, I will succumb to it much sooner than I would if I fight the bastard. My motto, "Never confuse the effort with the result." To live this motto, it is necessary to always keep the goal in mind.

By way of example, when I was in college, I used to run nine miles every day. Sometimes I would run a second time late at night. When I met Linda, I used to run from my parents' house to her parents' house so that I could see her. Running is a great way to become physically and mentally disciplined. When I was faced with a large hill to conquer, I would *never* look up at the top of that hill. Instead I would keep my head down, regulate my breathing, and look at the tiny stones in the asphalt. This allowed me to focus on my breathing etc. instead of the hill itself. All of a sudden, I realized I was over the top of that huge hill, and I didn't even know it. The point here is that each of us needs to fight cancer in his/her own way. *My* way is to apply the same concept of discipline to fighting cancer that I did when I was a runner. Instead of focusing on the constant treatments, appointments, injections, PET scans, MRI's, x-rays, biopsies, and all the other things that go with fighting this disease, it is imperative to have discipline and focus on the daily activities in our lives before the cancer was discovered. Remember, before diagnosis, it is probable that the cancer was there for some time, and no one knew it. In my case, the cancer started about three to five years *before* I was diagnosed. During that time, I was fishing, working out, doing my job, traveling with my wife, boating, etc. I never knew the cancer was there. But I still maintained these same activities after diagnosis, as I did before diagnosis. I strongly believe that normalcy helps a sick person heal. Therefore, it is important to keep daily life as normal as possible.

I know the chemo has side effects. Also, radiation has its issues as well. I get tired during the afternoon as a result of the chemo I am on. I take a twenty-minute snooze and then get back out to my activities. Again this helps a sick person heal. It also keeps your mind focused on life rather than the treatments and death. The mind is a powerhouse, and it is what determines much of what our bodies do. Therefore, it is so important to keep the mind focused on good rather than bad things. Remember, the glass must always be half full instead of half empty.

Some people can do this on their own while others need help. That is why family and friends, true friends, are so important. They become the catalyst that helps one promote healthy and positive thoughts for those who cannot do this on their own. Remember another thing: just because you may need family and friends to help you does not mean there is a weakness in you. Every one of us gets inspiration from different sources. Family and friends may be the way one person achieves positive thought while others seem to be able to handle things themselves. In my case, I seem to live on things that excite me. The ocean, which is the most inspirational part of nature that promotes for me positive feelings and thoughts, birds chirping early in the morning, trees blowing in the breeze, seeing small animals running about our yard, boats, great music, playing my musical instruments, etc. All contribute to my healthy thoughts.

Another part of my life that inspires me is by business. I created my practice from scratch and have maintained clients for over thirty years. Sure, some clients come and go, but the majority have been with me since the first five years of opening my practice. The business is like a child to me, and I still nurture it as I have in the past. I look forward to going to work in the mornings as much as I always did, and this helps me heal too. Everyone needs to find what inspires themselves. One other major inspirational driver for me is my upbringing. I believe that the way my parents brought us up, particularly my mother, has a great deal to do with my positive thought and the "drive" I seem to have. I mentioned this earlier in this writing, but I will mention it again because it is the foundation that drives all the other things that inspire me.

My wife is also inspirational to me. Her very existence gives me a reason to always move forward. Linda is the most important and loved person in my life, and *that* love also inspires me to always move forward. I have visions of the day we can enjoy our lives without the need for chemo treatments, radiation, MRIs, etc., and all the side effects resulting from them. So keep on moving forward and find those things in your life that inspire you. You should find them by those things you enjoyed as a child. The child is still in each of us; most seem to forget this as they go through the years.

Emergency Room Visit

On Friday, August 7, 2020, I was at Brigham for my radiation treatments. On the way, I sent a message to my primary care doctor of an event that took place the afternoon before. I was with my wife, and we were running errands. We were laughing and having a great time when suddenly I lost my bearings and found myself dazed and confused. I did not say anything to Linda as I did not want to alarm her. I explained to my doctor the circumstances, and she demanded I walk over to the emergency room immediately after my treatments. I complied.

All sorts of tests were performed from COVID-19 test to CT scans of my neck and head. Nothing was found. During the visit, I was fortunate enough to have a nurse assigned to me who has been at the hospital for many years and had vast experience. It turns out that she has a place in Naples not far from ours. We exchanged telephone numbers and vowed to keep in touch so that we could all get together when in Naples at the same time.

It appears that I was both exhausted from the traveling and working during the week and dehydrated as well. It did not help that I was working in the yard moving boulders the size of my torso that past Sunday, and that Saturday we went kayaking the whole day. I recall being somewhat tired that day, and when lifting the rocks, I found I would get a little dizzy too. Guess I was overdoing it for several days. I promised the doctors I would refrain from such activities while on the radiation treatments and the chemo for the prostate cancer. We still did work in the yard, but I was doing *much* lighter work. I did, however, continue to comply with these requests because, while I am always on the go, I simply do not want to make matters worse. Having rested for two weekends, I did feel much better.

Radiation Complete

On September 15, 2020, I received my last radiation treatment for the prostate cancer. I started in July and received forty-four such treatments over sixty-two days. I would hike to Boston every Monday through Friday. The only weekday I had off was Labor Day. My PSA is nearly nonexistent and my testosterone as well. It seems these treatments eradicated that cancer. One down and one more to go!

The plan now is to monitor the PSA every few months and hope it doesn't rise again. If it does, I cannot have surgery because I had the radiation. I am unsure what will be done at that point, so I am praying the PSA stays very low. Also, now I am to begin to address the first two cancers again. Dr. Laubach has set up tests to measure the light chains and hopefully they have not risen. If they are down, he stated he would hold off with any maintenance chemo for a short period of months to give my body a rest. Hopefully, with the maintenance chemo; once I start that again, will keep me in remission until a cure is found.

If, however, the light chain cells had risen while off the chemo for this cancer during the radiation session, I will need to go back on the full chemo regimen. And depending on the level of the light chains and the ratio of the kappa and lambda cells, it will affect the length of time I will be on these treatments. My hope, of course, is to not have to take this course of action. However, if I had to, I certainly will proceed as I have from the start: work every day, keep my life as normal as possible, and do the things I did before cancer.

I received the test results of the light chains and lambda and kappa on Friday, September 11, 2020. Things looked steady and within the range of normal. I was delighted. I actually started to cry from relief. I stated to Linda that I will hear from Dr. Jacob Laubach this weekend. Sure enough, he called at 10:00 p.m. Sunday, September 13, 2020. He too was delighted, and we agreed that we would *not* begin any treatments now but would take a break to allow my body to rest, and we would test again second week in November.

I was thrilled! I so look forward to spending a full day at the office, which I have not been able to do for sixty-two days. But for now, the three cancers are as follows: prostate is eradicated, multiple myeloma does not show up at this point in my blood work or the readings from the blood, amyloidosis is currently in remission. Dr. Laubach and I both know that the amyloid cancer cells will rear their ugly head again. It could be tomorrow or next year, but they will become active again. Until the research doctors come up with a cure to mitigate the ability of these cells to multiply, I will have to monitor them on a monthly basis. I will do that. And when I am required to once again receive treatments to knock them down into remission again, I will do my best to keep the positive attitude and continue to move forward, always looking to the goal line.

Final Thoughts

Remember, I truly believe that normalcy helps to heal. Cancer poses so many different and unexpected effects on the body that sometimes it is hard to keep focused. I have many things in my life to help keep me focused: my beautiful wife, Linda; our boat, which is my inspiration as *I love* being on the ocean; our Naples home; my practice; the many friends and aunts, uncles, cousins, and other family members who proved to me that they are true to me. So many have kept in touch with me through this entire process, my clients who stood by me and continue to do so. And God, because without my belief in him, I just don't know where I would be.

If you have cancer, don't baby yourself. Move and keep going. As hard as it is, it is important to maintain a healthy lifestyle so that you can keep a positive attitude. If you are a caregiver of someone who is sick, whether it be cancer or any other such illness, keep your loved one moving and *never* let up. Sometimes the patient will not feel strong enough to get out of bed but *you* have to push the person. Once up, things get easier.

Cancer patients have something in common that those without such a disease simply cannot fully understand. We eventually become very much in tune to our inner self. We also don't want to waste any time because, while we know everyone will die, we seem to be faced with a deadline that we cannot measure, but we know it is probably going to be sooner than what time we would have if we did not have cancer.

It is crucial to keep focused and moving forward. Further, never fall backward, fall forward. At least you would have made some progress. That is important. You know what you can do, and you need to do it. Stay focused and always look to things that inspired you from an early age. For me, this is nature, the ocean, music, etc. These keep me grounded. Find those things that inspire you and never lose faith. Stay grounded, and may God bless you for many years to come.

About The Cover

The cover of this book is a photograph I took of the Watch Hill Lighthouse in Watch Hill, Rhode Island, when I was a commercial fisherman. I wanted to use this photograph because the fog represents the "fog" of sickness while the lit lens represents the "light" one must keep his/her focus on when fighting cancer or any other disease. Often times it is difficult to keep focused on that light at the end of the tunnel because of all the "fog" life and sickness throws at us. I often look at this and other photographs I took over the years while on the water to inspire me to never lose sight of that shining beacon.

About the Author

T he author is a certified public accountant operating his
practice in Smithfield, Rhode
Island. A 1983 graduate of Bryant
College (now Bryant University)
in Smithfield, Rhode Island, he
attended Community College of
Rhode Island before transferring to
Bryant College. In his practice, Joe
is an adviser to numerous small busi-
nesses in various states. He operates
with the motto "Treat every client as
if he/she is the only one."

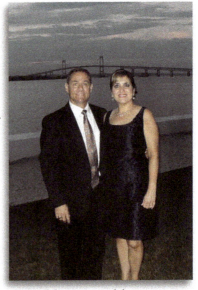

Joe is also a United States Coast
Guard–licensed captain holding a
100 Gross Ton Master license. He is an avid boater and loves to visit
ports of call with his wife, Linda, throughout New England and New
York. Boating is his passion, and for many years, he was a commercial
fisherman. He no longer fishes commercially but devotes time to con-
servation efforts and refuses to kill any fish from the ocean.

Due to his need to constantly monitor his cancer cells, Joe has
no plans of leaving Rhode Island and wants to be close to Dana-
Farber in Boston, Massachusetts, for these tests. However, Joe and
Linda enjoy spending time in Naples, Florida. They spend time with
friends there and love being on the water. Shopping on 5th Avenue is
also a staple for the couple.

CPSIA information can be obtained
at www.ICGtesting.com
Printed in the USA
BVHW090015280721
613018BV00021B/1528